Dr Sarah Brewer graduated from Cambridge University as a Natural Scientist in 1980. She went on to study medicine at Cambridge Clinical School, where she qualified as a doctor in 1983. Although her first love is medicine, her major passion is writing. She is pursuing a career in medical journalism to successfully combine the two.

Sarah writes regularly for a wide variety of newspapers and magazines including *Marie Clare*, *Prime*, *The Lady* and *The Daily Express*. She has written numerous books including: *The Daily Telegraph Encyclopedia of Vitamins, Minerals and Herbal Supplements* (Constable & Robinson), *Eat to Beat I.B.S.* (Thorsons), *Total Detox Plan* (Carlton Books) and *Pregnancy the Natural Way* (Souvenir Press Ltd).

PLANNING A BABY?

How to prepare for a healthy
pregnancy and give your baby
the best possible start

Dr Sarah Brewer

Vermilion
LONDON

5 7 9 10 8 6 4

First published in the United Kingdom in 1995 by Optima
First published in 1998 by Vermilion

This revised edition published in the United Kingdom in 2004 by Vermilion
an imprint of Ebury Press
Random House Group Ltd
Random House
20 Vauxhall Bridge Road
London SW1V 2SA

Random House Australia (Pty) Ltd
20 Alfred Street, Milsons Point, Sydney
New South Wales 2061, Australia

Random House New Zealand Limited
18 Poland Road, Glenfield
Auckland 10, New Zealand

Random House (Pty) Limited
Isle of Houghton, Corner of Boundary Road & Carse O'Gowrie,
Houghton 2198, South Africa

The Random House Group Limited Reg. No. 954009
www.randomhouse.co.uk

Papers used by Vermilion are natural, recyclable products made
from wood grown in sustainable forests.

A CIP catalogue record for this book is available from the British Library

ISBN 9780091898489 (from January 2007)
ISBN 009189848X

Typeset by SX Composing DTP, Rayleigh, Essex

Printed and bound in Great Britain by
Mackays of Chatham plc, Chatham, Kent

Contents

Introduction

Deciding to start a family is a time of great joy, adventure and hope. It is also a time of apprehension. Are we fertile? How long will I take to conceive? When should we make love? What dietary changes should we make? Question after question is raised – of which perhaps the most important is – will I be able to produce a healthy baby?

It's estimated that between 60 and 70 per cent of babies born in the Western world are planned, allowing plenty of opportunity for advanced preparation. By following a pre-conceptual care programme, and ensuring both you and your partner are in the peak of health, you can maximise your chances of success.

The most critical time of a baby's development is the first four weeks of gestation – often before the mother is even aware that she is pregnant. Recent studies suggest the development of coronary heart disease, stroke or diabetes in later years is linked to growth failure in the first few weeks of life. If a baby is under-nourished at this critical time, it may become programmed to develop high blood pressure, blood clotting disorders, or abnormal glucose, insulin and cholesterol metabolism in middle age.

You can never adopt a healthy diet and lifestyle too soon where pregnancy and your future offspring are concerned. You should start at least three months – and preferably six – before you try to conceive.

Research shows that following a pre-conceptual care programme greatly increases the chance of successfully conceiving a healthy baby, especially if a women takes pre-conceptual folic acid supplements and avoids cigarette smoking (active or passive) and excessive alcohol intake.

Pre-conceptual care is just as important for the future father as it is for the mother. It takes 100 days to produce a sperm, from the first division of its primitive germ cell until ejaculation. That's 100 crucial days in which, if properly nurtured, sperm will flourish. Dietary and lifestyle carelessness can cause irreparable damage that may project into future generations.

More women are now having babies in their thirties than in their twenties, mostly through choice in delaying motherhood and establishing their career first. Female fertility naturally decreases with age, however, and it will take an average of six months (and sometimes as long as two years) to conceive at the age of 35 compared with two to three months at the age of 25.

I first wrote *Planning a Baby* as a means of researching pre-conceptual care before starting a family myself. I was amazed at how much information was available in the medical literature, but how little was available for the general public. Since writing the first edition of this book, pre-conceptual care has come on in leaps and bounds, with folic acid supplements now routinely recommended, and many GP surgeries and hospitals offering pre-conceptual counselling. I followed the information in my book myself and was thrilled to become pregnant the first time round, at the age of 38, during the first month of trying. It took six months to conceive my second pregnancy, at the age of 41, but I was delighted to discover I was expecting twins. One of the advantages (?!) of postponing motherhood into later life is that the chance of twins does increase.

Best of luck with starting your own family – one of the most exciting adventures on which any couple can embark.

Dr Sarah Brewer

PART I
For future mums

The female reproductive system

The female menstrual cycle

The hormonal fluctuations that occur throughout a female's menstrual cycle trigger changes in the ovaries, uterus (womb) and cervix. Understanding these changes is important during the pre-conceptual programme. They can be used to:

- Follow the natural fertility awareness method of contraception while preparing for future pregnancy (see pages 16–20).
- Maximise your chances of conception once you've decided it's time to try.

The uterine cycle

The female menstrual cycle is the periodic preparation of the endometrium (womb lining) for implantation of a fertilised egg.

The length of the menstrual cycle is variable. In some women it lasts 21 days or less; in others, 35 days between the start of each period is normal. A regular 28-day cycle, usually considered the 'norm', is in fact enjoyed by only 12 per cent of females. Menstruation itself usually lasts from one to eight days, with the majority of women experiencing bleeding for three to five days.

The most fertile time of the month lasts for the six days up to, and including, the day of ovulation. The time of ovulation varies, although it is usually said to occur around 14 days before your next period is due. New research shows that the timing of ovulation is highly unpredictable, however, even in women whose cycles are regular. When around 700 menstrual cycles were assessed among 221 women trying to conceive, only 30 per cent had their fertile phase entirely between day 10 and day 17 of the cycle (the first day of the last period is counted as day 1). Most women reached their fertile window earlier, and others much later. At least 10 per cent of women were fertile on any given day between days 6 and 21, and up to 6 per cent were potentially fertile even on the day their next period was due.

Control of the menstrual cycle

Cervical mucus changes, the waxing and waning of the endometrium and the development of the ovarian follicle are all synchronised by the female hormones.

The key to the cycle is the corpus luteum – the collapsed follicle from which the egg was recently released. If pregnancy occurs, this remains functional (by receiving feedback hormones from the developing placenta), the endometrium is maintained and menstruation prevented. If pregnancy does not occur, the corpus luteum stops making oestrogen and progesterone. This triggers menstruation and also the release of FSH (follicle stimulating hormone) and LH (luteinising hormone) from the pituitary gland. These in turn trigger the development of a new batch of ovarian follicles (eggs). As ovarian follicles start to develop under the influence of pituitary hormones (see page 10) they secrete oestrogen.

Oestrogen from the developing follicles stimulates the endometrium, which then thickens. Endometrial glands become elongated and straight and grow rapidly during the first two weeks of the menstrual cycle. This is called the *proliferative* (or follicular) phase. After ovulation, blood vessels rapidly grow into the thickened endometrium. It becomes soft and spongy under the influence of the hormone progesterone, which, along with oestrogen, is secreted by the empty ovarian follicle (corpus luteum).

The endometrium reaches a maximum thickness of around 5 mm. Its glands become coiled and tortuous and start to secrete a clear, nourishing fluid, which will provide the fertilised egg with nutrients before and after its implants. This part of the menstrual cycle is therefore called the *secretory* phase.

If pregnancy occurs, the empty ovarian follicle (corpus luteum) is triggered to continue secreting oestrogen and progesterone by HCG (human chorionic gonadotrophin) from the developing placenta. This prevents further shedding of the endometrium until after the baby is born.

If pregnancy does not occur, the corpus luteum deteriorates after ten days and stops making hormones around four days before the next period starts.

Arteries supplying the endometrium with blood go into spasm and the lining thins and starts to disintegrate. The outer two thirds of the endometrium are then shed as a menstrual period – almost exactly fourteen days after ovulation occurred. All but the deep layers of the endometrium are cast off and a new cycle now begins.

Anovulatory cycles

In some cycles, ovulation fails. This is most common during the first eighteen months of puberty and again as the menopause approaches.

When ovulation fails, there is no corpus luteum to secrete the progesterone necessary for the secretory phase of the menstrual cycle. Oestrogens from the ovary continue to cause growth, however, and the proliferative phase of the cycle carries on.

Soon, the endometrium becomes thick enough to outgrow its blood supply and it starts to break down, triggering a menstrual bleed. The time it takes for bleeding to occur is variable but is usually less than 28 days from the onset of the previous period. Bleeding also varies from scanty to profuse.

Cervical mucus cycle

Throughout a normal menstrual cycle, changes occur in mucus secreted by the cervix. During the proliferative phase of the cycle, the hormone oestrogen encourages the production of mucus which is thin and alkaline (non acidic). This type of mucus is ideal for the survival and easy penetration of sperm. Mucus becomes increasingly

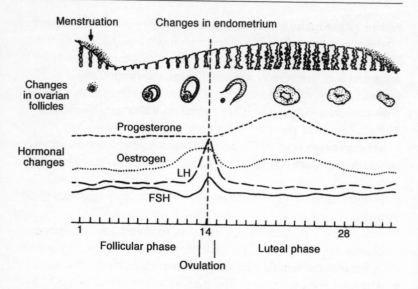

The female menstrual cycle

fluid, slippery and elastic until ovulation occurs. At this time, a drop
of cervical mucus can be stretched into a long, thin thread up to 15
cm (6 inches) long. The molecules in the mucus are well aligned and
it is easy for sperm to swim through. (See also page 17.)

Within a day of ovulation, the cervical mucus suddenly changes
in character under the influence of the hormone progesterone. It
becomes thick, sticky, scant and hostile to sperm. It is inelastic and
the molecules within are entangled like a tight mesh, making it
difficult for sperm to swim through.

Similar hormone-related changes affect saliva, and examining
these changes through a pocket-sized microscope (Calista, see page
19) is the latest method for predicting ovulation.

Oogenesis

The female reproductive cells, the ova or eggs, are made in a
process known as oogenesis. This differs from the formation of
sperm (spermatogenesis) in several important ways:

- Unlike the male, in whom spermatogenesis starts at puberty, the major part of oogenesis occurs in the female foetus before birth. The final stage of the development of each egg only occurs just before it is released during ovulation.
- Each primitive germ cell (spermatogonium) in the male continues dividing and can produce as many as 512 sperm. Each primitive germ cell (oogonium) in the female only produces two eggs as a result of two unequal divisions. The smaller product of each division is cast off and absorbed as waste.
- It takes around 380 cell divisions to form a sperm, but only 23 to make an egg.
- Each human female is born with her full complement of eggs. Unlike the male, who continues making new sperm for the rest of his life, the female cannot make new eggs after she is born.
- After puberty, women release eggs at a rate of one (occasionally more) per month. The male releases millions of sperm per ejaculation.
- Sperm production continues into advanced old age. The monthly release of eggs stops once a female reaches the menopause.

These differences have important consequences for pre-conceptual care. As it takes around 100 days to make a batch of sperm, a man can follow a careful pre-conceptual care programme for at least three months before trying for a baby. By providing optimal conditions for his sperm to grow, he can be fairly confident they are present in peak quality and quantity (see page 185).

By the time a woman wants to start a family, her eggs may already be 16 to 48 years old. As eggs get older, the risk of deterioration increases. That's the main reason why increasing maternal age is associated with an increased risk of having offspring with genetic abnormalities such as Down's Syndrome (see page 259). So pre-conceptual care for the future mother is aimed more at improving her general health for the nine months of pregnancy ahead, rather than dramatically improving the quality of released eggs.

Even so, it is useful to understand how eggs are released each month. By seeing how this fits into the menstrual cycle, it's possible to calculate the most fertile part of the month.

How the ovaries and eggs develop

The ovaries start developing during the first few weeks of foetal life. The outer layer of the ovary (cortex) contains primitive germ cells called oogonia. These are equivalent to the spermatogonia from which the male's sperm arise.

The oogonia rapidly mature and develop. By the third month after conception, they undergo a series of normal divisions and multiply to form around seven million primary oocytes. Each primary oocyte has the same number of genes, divided into 46 chromosomes, as every other cell in the body.

The oocytes now enter a specialised form of cell division (meiosis) in which half the usual number of chromosomes – 23 – go to each daughter cell.

Meiosis is a two-stage process. During the first stage, the chromosomes double up and pair off. The chromosomes exchange random blocks of genes within each pair. After exchanging genetic material, the paired chromosomes separate to either end of the cell ready for the oocyte to divide again.

At this stage, development of the egg suddenly stops before this division is complete. The egg is virtually frozen in time and will not complete this division until just before ovulation – some 10 to 50 years after the process was started.

In the female oocytes (unlike a male's spermatocytes) this division, when it does finally occur *just before ovulation*, is unequal. One daughter cell gets most of the cell material (cytoplasm) of the parent cell. The smaller offspring cell (called the first polar body) fragments and disappears.

After ovulation, the new daughter oocyte now contains a different mix of genes, arranged in a different order on the 46 chromosomes, than are found in the woman's other body cells. It immediately enters the second stage of meiosis.

The chromosomes split and half of each one separates to either end of the cell. The egg now starts to divide unequally again. This time, one daughter cell takes half the usual number of chromosomes

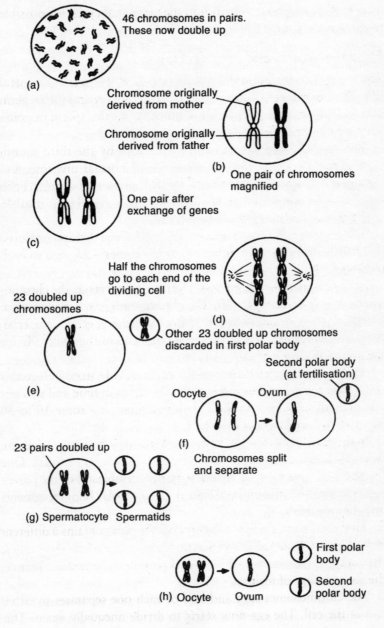

(a) 46 chromosomes in pairs. These now double up

(b) One pair of chromosomes magnified

Chromosome originally derived from mother

Chromosome originally derived from father

(c) One pair after exchange of genes

(d) Half the chromosomes go to each end of the dividing cell

(e) 23 doubled up chromosomes

Other 23 doubled up chromosomes discarded in first polar body

Second polar body (at fertilisation)

(f) Oocyte   Ovum

Chromosomes split and separate

(g) 23 pairs doubled up

Spermatocyte   Spermatids

(h) Oocyte   Ovum

First polar body

Second polar body

Meiosis

(23 instead of 46) and most of the cell material. The other product of division, containing half the genetic material and very little cytoplasm, will again be cast off as waste. This final division, like the first, is frozen just before completion and is only properly finished when a sperm penetrates the egg. At this stage, the unwanted half of genetic material is cast off as the second polar body and the fertilised egg proceeds to develop into a new individual.

As a result of the swapping and splitting up of genes that occurs during meiosis, each egg contains a unique set of genes – a random half selection from the primitive parent cell from which it originated. Some eggs may have a similar selection of genes to other eggs – accounting for family similarities between future brothers and sisters – but no two will ever be identical.

Ovarian follicles

The eight million primary oocytes within the ovarian cortex are each surrounded by a single layer of flattened cells. These cells plus the immature egg inside are known as the primordial follicles.

The cells surrounding each follicle are also important and are known as granulosa cells. They are full of tiny granules rich in cholesterol which will eventually be converted into female hormones.

During the fifth and sixth months of foetal life, many primordial follicles start to break up. A five-month-old female foetus contains about seven million eggs. By the time of birth, this number falls to two million and by the time of puberty, only 40,000 to 400,000 primordial follicles remain. The rest have slowly degenerated and become re-absorbed.

No new eggs are ever formed after birth – when we talk about making eggs, we mean maturation of egg cells (primary oocytes) already present in the ovary.

Ovarian changes at puberty

At puberty, the ovaries are switched on by two hormones secreted in the pituitary gland at the base of the brain. These hormones are follicle stimulating hormone (FSH) and luteinising hormone (LH). They are the same hormones that, in the male, trigger the production of sperm in the testicles.

In the female, FSH triggers the production and development of several ovarian follicles at the start of each cycle. As well as growing in size, the granulosa cells surrounding the follicle start to secrete oestrogen hormone. Blood levels of oestrogen start to rise.

In humans, one follicle starts to grow more rapidly on about the sixth day of development and continues to outpace the rest. It produces increasing amounts of oestrogen which has a dampening effect on the production of hormones in the pituitary gland in the brain. As a result, blood levels of FSH fall slightly. When this happens, the non-dominant follicles stop growing and start to regress. Only the dominant follicle continues to grow because it has matured enough to respond to the falling levels of FSH.

It is not yet known how this follicle is singled out for development. If women are given highly purified pituitary hormones (FSH and LH) as a fertility treatment, many follicles continue to develop, hence the increased incidence of a multiple pregnancy.

The maturing follicle

As a follicle starts to mature, a fluid-filled cavity forms around the egg cell inside. The egg becomes suspended at the top of a hillock of cells within the fluid and the follicle continues to swell. It is now known as a Graafian follicle after the scientist who first described it.

By the time of ovulation after 10 to 14 days of growth, the Graafian follicle measures 1.8–2.6 cm across and bulges from the surface of the ovary. During this process, the immature egg inside the follicle also enlarges. Granulosa cells secrete a thick protective coating around the egg – rather like chunky egg white – which will form a future barrier against sperm so that only one can successfully penetrate the egg.

In the few hours before ovulation, the chromosomes within the egg cell that first started to divide during the third month of foetal life are finally arranged correctly within the nucleus. The egg now immediately enters its second meiotic division and then stops, almost frozen in time. This division will only be completed upon fertilisation by a sperm. At that time, as already described above, an unequal division occurs and half the genetic material is extruded as the second polar body.

At ovulation, the follicle ruptures and a blob of jelly containing the egg oozes out. Some women notice mid-cycle pain (known as Mittelschmertz) at around this time due to pressure within the swollen egg follicle. The empty follicle now collapses and forms a yellow cyst known as the corpus luteum. This secretes the female hormones oestrogen and progesterone. Progesterone prevents menstruation and the development of other ovarian follicles during the remainder of the monthly cycle. For the next 10 days, the corpus luteum swells and becomes as large as 2 cm across.

If a pregnancy occurs, the corpus luteum continues its secretory role and maintains early pregnancy by preventing menstruation. After the third month of pregnancy, the placenta takes over all hormone production and the corpus luteum fades away. If pregnancy doesn't occur, the corpus luteum degenerates after about 10 days. This triggers menstruation and the start of a new cycle.

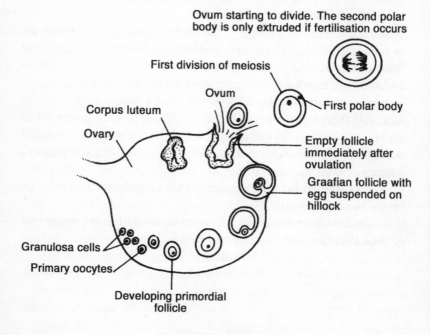

The maturing follicle

It is estimated that only 300 to 500 ovarian follicles come to full maturity and release eggs during a woman's reproductive life. If she uses a hormonal method of contraception such as the combined oral contraceptive pill, ovulation is suppressed and a woman may release fewer than 100 eggs during her lifetime.

The released egg

As a rule, only one egg is released each month in humans. Contrary to popular belief, an egg is not released from each ovary on alternate months. There doesn't seem to be a pattern and eggs are released from the two ovaries in an irregular and unpredictable sequence. Some women regularly ovulate two or more eggs, which increases the chance of twins, triplets or higher multiple births. Interestingly, egg cells seem to become less receptive in later life to the signals telling them to stop developing, so that two or more eggs may continue maturing and are released at ovulation. As a result, women who conceive in their forties are more likely to produce twins because of this phenomenon.

Immediately after ovulation, the fresh egg is sucked into the end of a Fallopian tube. This is wrapped round the ovary at the site of follicular rupture. The inside surface of the Fallopian tube is covered with tiny hair-like projections (cilia), which beat rapidly to set up eddy currents. These suck the newly released egg into the tube and then carry it downwards on what has been described as the ciliary escalator. Fluid currents and contraction of the muscular walls of the Fallopian tubes also contribute to the egg's downward journey.

It's not known how long the egg remains fertilisable within the tube – but it is probably for only a short period of around one day. If fertilisation does not occur while the egg is within the upper end of the Fallopian tube, it starts to degenerate.

2

Contraception

Family planning is an essential part of reproductive health and pre-conceptual care. In ideal circumstances, effective contraception allows women to choose whether to have children, how many and when. You will need to decide:

- Whether to continue with your current method of contraception.
- If discontinuing your current method, when to do so.
- Whether to switch to a natural family planning technique.
- Whether to switch to a barrier method of contraception.
- When to come off the Pill – probably the most commonly asked question.

If pre-conceptual care is to be most effective, it is essential that the future parents can rely on their chosen method of contraception. It must be:

- Safe – both for them and their future offspring.
- Effective.
- Reliable.
- Readily reversible.
- Easy to use.
- It must not interfere too much with the spontaneity and pleasure of making love.

Most women who are currently using a hormonal method of contraception or the coil (IUCD – intra-uterine contraceptive device) will wish to change either to natural, fertility awareness methods of contraception or to a barrier method. Only you can choose which method is right for you. Personal advice is available from your doctor or a family planning specialist. Useful addresses are included in the back of the book (see pages 272–283).

In order to answer most of your questions, the following chapter provides information on:

• The various methods of contraception available.
• How they are used and how they work.
• Whether they are suitable during pre-conceptual care.

Failure rates of various methods

Most contraception failures are caused by human error such as forgetting to take a Pill, tearing a condom or removing a diaphragm too early.

The following table shows how effective various methods of contraception are, giving the typical pregnancy rates during the first year of use. The figures given are failures per 100 women, which in effect is the same as a percentage failure rate.

Method	Typical failure rate
No contraception	85
Withdrawal	19
Natural fertility awareness methods	Up to 23
Fertility awareness computer (Persona)	6 or more
Diaphragm/cap	Up to 18
Spermicides alone	25
Male condom	Up to 15
Female condom	Up to 15
Coil (IUCD)	1 to 2

Progestogen coil (intra-uterine system)	< 1
Progestogen implant	< 1
Depot progestogen injection	< 1
Combined Pill	< 1–3 or more
Mini Pill	< 1–4 or more
Contraceptive patch	< 1
Female sterilisation	< 1
Male sterilisation	< 1
Emergency contraceptive Pill	Up to 4
Emergency contraceptive IUCD	Up to 2

Natural family planning methods

Withdrawal

The withdrawal method is undoubtedly the oldest method of contraception.

If practised carefully, it is surprisingly effective. Some studies show no difference in failure rates between the withdrawal method and barrier methods such as the diaphragm. Although there are many better methods of contraception available, withdrawal is better than nothing and may be the method of choice for some couples during the pre-conceptual care period.

Fertility awareness

Fertility awareness or 'natural' methods of contraception involve monitoring physical changes that occur throughout the menstrual cycle to predict the most fertile period. Unprotected sex is then avoided during this time, and you may either abstain from sex or use another method of contraception such as a condom. It requires proper training and a thorough understanding of the method, as recent research suggests that the timing of ovulation is not as predictable as previously thought. At least 10 per cent of women seem to be fertile on any given day between days 6 and 21 of their cycle, and up to 6 per cent are potentially fertile even on the day their next period was due. Fertility awareness can be as effective as barrier methods of contraception with careful use – failure rates are usually quoted as ranging from 2 per cent to 20 per cent. A large population study in the US, however, found that 9 to 16 per cent of married women and 21 to 23 per cent of single women using natural birth control became pregnant within a year even though they did not intend to. Because no chemicals are involved, because it is a 'natural' method that helps you predict when you are more fertile once you are ready to start a family, this is a popular contraceptive choice during the pre-conceptual period.

Fertility awareness involves monitoring body changes that help you predict when ovulation has occurred. As some women seem to ovulate at different times in each cycle, and as a few women seem to ovulate more than once in a cycle, its reliability is difficult to assess.

The changes that may be monitored include:

- Body temperature: Immediately after ovulation, body temperature drops slightly and then rises by 0.2–0.4 degrees Centigrade. It then stays high until the next period starts. Women are advised to take their core body temperature using a special fertility (expanded-scale) thermometer on waking and before getting out of bed. Results are plotted daily on a chart.
- Cervical mucus: Before ovulation, cervical mucus becomes increasingly fluid and slippery due to the effects of oestrogen hormone. It has a consistency similar to egg white and may be drawn between two fingers to a length of several centimetres. The alignment of mucus molecules allows sperm to swim through it easily and survive for a relatively long time (see page 6). Immediately after ovulation, cervical mucus becomes thick and sticky under the influence of progesterone hormone. It then becomes more hostile to sperm and, because the mucus molecules are entangled, sperm cannot swim through as easily. The quantity, fluidity, glossiness, transparency and elasticity of cervical mucus is observed on each visit to the bathroom. You

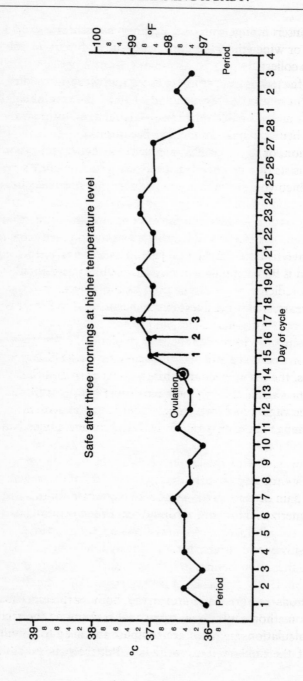

Typical ovulatory temperature chart

can either insert a finger into the vagina to assess dryness or moistness, or wipe yourself with toilet tissue and examine the mucus you collect.

- Saliva: Is affected by the presence of oestrogen and luteinising hormone during the fertile days of your cycle. By examining dried saliva under a pocket microscope (sold as Calista) you can time when you make love either as a form of contraception, or to maximise your chances of conception. Calista consists of a powerful, pocket-sized, backlit microscope through which you examine a sample of saliva. You just place a little saliva on the optical block and wait for it to dry. Your dried saliva will show a dotted pattern on non-ovulating days, or a clear fern-like pattern that indicates ovulation is imminent and you have reached your fertile peak. Clinical trials show that Calista is 98 per cent accurate and – unlike urine-based ovulation predictor kits – can be used month after month for over two years, making it a less expensive method to use. It is available from most pharmacies, and from www.ecobrands.co.uk.
- The position and texture of the cervix: As the fertile phase approaches, the cervix becomes softer, pouts open and rises higher in the vagina. During the infertile phase, the cervix sits lower in the vagina and feels firm, rubbery and dry with a closed opening. These changes are less easy to detect once you have had a child.
- Mood changes.
- Mid-cycle spotting of blood.
- Mid-cycle pain occurring 24–48 hours before ovulation (Mittelschmertz): This is due to distension of the ovarian capsule.
- Breast sensitivity.
- Acne and other skin changes.

Natural methods require commitment by both partners. Those choosing this method must receive personal training as the techniques and calculations involved are complex and need to be fully understood if the method is to work as effectively as possible.

Monitoring must occur throughout the menstrual cycle, and you must be careful not to confuse cervical mucus with semen or spermicide so the wrong characteristics are noticed.

Persona

Persona makes natural fertility awareness more effective. It involves dip-testing your urine on eight days of your monthly cycle (16 days in the first month) and inserting the test stick into a small, hand-held analyser. This measures levels of natural hormones in your urine to assess when you are most at risk of pregnancy. Failure rates are around 6 per cent or greater depending on how properly it is used, and how rigorously you avoid unsafe sex on unsafe days.

The diaphragm

The diaphragm covers the cervix and upper vagina, acting as a female barrier contraceptive. It is kept in place by the action of the vaginal muscles, the pubic bone and by a spring within its rim. Sizes range from 5 to 10 cm in diameter.

Fitting by a trained family planning specialist is required. If a woman's weight changes by more than half a stone (3 kg) it is essential that the diaphragm's fit is rechecked. A diaphragm can be inserted either way up, but maintains the correct position more readily if inserted dome upwards.

As the upper third of the vagina balloons during intercourse, semen often gets past and spermicidal agents are essential. Failure rates when used with a spermicide range from 2 to 15 per cent.

A diaphragm should not be left in place for longer than 24 hours. This both encourages infection and gives a theoretical risk of pressure damage to vaginal walls.

The cap

The cap is smaller than a diaphragm. It looks rather like a thimble and fits directly over the cervix. The new silicone version (Oves) is most popular today.

Spermicides

Spermicides are substances which physically or chemically immobilise or destroy sperm on prolonged contact. They are available as aerosol foams, jellies, creams, impregnated films, pessaries or sponges which are inserted into the vagina before making love.

Spermicides are not recommended for use without a barrier method of contraception, but in those studies where sole use has occurred, failure rates vary between 4 and 25 per cent.

Spermicides contain both an inert carrier base and an active agent. Water-soluble bases are preferable as mineral oil-based agents weaken the latex rubber of condoms and diaphragms by up to 95 per cent within fifteen minutes.

Active spermicidal ingredients include:

- Surface-active agents, e.g. nonoxynol-9.
- Enzyme inhibitors.
- Some anti-bacterial agents.
- Acids, e.g. lactic acid.
- Local anaesthetics which affect sperm cell membranes.

Studies suggest that some spermicides are protective against sexually transmissible diseases. Nonoxynol-9 is active against Neisseria gonorrhoea, chlamydia, herpes simplex virus, human immuno-deficiency virus (HIV), trichomonas vaginalis and candida (thrush).

There is no evidence that fertilisation with a sperm damaged through exposure to spermicidal agents, or inadvertent use during pregnancy, might result in a foetal abnormality.

The male condom

Male condoms are made from vulcanised latex rubber, or from polyurethane, which has the advantages of being twice as strong as latex, thinner and non-allergenic.

Condoms provide a physical barrier so that sperm do not enter the female reproductive tract. They are most effective when used with a spermicidal cream or gel. Apart from protecting against any spilled sperm, this provides extra lubrication so the condom is less likely to burst than when used dry. It is important to use only a water-based lubricant, as petroleum jelly and mineral oils such as baby oil weaken latex rubber (they do not harm polyurethane condoms, however). Condoms also help to protect against sexually transmissible infections.

Condoms are available non-lubricated, lubricated with the spermicide nonoxynol-9, or with a non-spermicidal lubricant (sk-70) for those with allergies. Condoms are available in two standard widths in the UK – 52 mm and 49 mm. The selection is broadened by the choice of several different contours to provide optimum fit and sensitivity. The table opposite acts as a guide to the different shapes to choose from.

Improving sensitivity

Many men are unaware that advances in condom technology can improve sensitivity. Shaped condoms, for example, can provide extra comfort, a feeling of roominess, or a snugger fit which many men prefer – once they've tried it – to the traditional straight up-and-down designs. Gel charging can also boost sensitivity to give a more natural sensation – almost as if a condom is not being used.

Gel charging involves putting a small amount of water-based lubricating gel (around one teaspoon – 5 ml) inside the condom before putting it on in the usual way. It helps to warm the tube of gel in warm water first so it isn't too cold. During love-making, the gel warms further and liquefies to provide extra stimulation.

Gel charging should only be tried with a shaped condom – contoured or flared – which retains the gel more easily and makes slipping less likely during use.

Protection against infections

Using a condom can reduce the risk of catching gonorrhoea, NSU (chlamydia), trichomonas, herpes, hepatitis or HIV if your partner is infected, but are not foolproof. The spermicide nonoxynol-9 adds to the protection as it can kill some infections in the same way that it kills sperm. By reducing the risk of sexually transmitted

Straight	Same width up and down.	For men who are used to the traditional shape.
Flared	Wide head, tapered at tip.	For extra comfort; condom feels larger and less restrictive; useful for men who usually find condoms too tight.
Contoured: wide head and neck	Anatomically shaped for a better fit – flared over glans and snug below.	For improved sensitivity and comfort; helps to prevent slippage; excellent starter condom.
Contoured: wide head and smaller neck	Anatomically shaped for better fit over glans. Width at base of penis 49 mm for a closer fit.	Helps to prevent slippage; a closer and firmer fit for those who require it.
Textured	Condoms possess ribs or dots.	Designed for increased friction and heightened sensation. Use with water-based lubricant to prevent soreness. Not suitable for oral sex.
Ultra-thin	Slightly thinner latex.	For greater sensitivity; only for experienced users.
Super-strong	Thicker latex (e.g. 50% thicker than normal).	For extra-vigorous sex.
Non-spermicide lubricant		For use if either partner is allergic to spermicides.
With integral applicator		For those who prefer a no-touch technique, who have difficulty applying a normal condom, or who regularly burst condoms on opening the packet or donning the condom.
Polyurethane		For improved sensitivity and for those who are allergic to latex.

infections, using condoms also reduces the risk of pelvic inflammatory disease in women and may reduce the risk of cervical cancer.

When used correctly, condoms have a method failure rate of 2
to 5 per cent per year. However, incorrect use, and the risk of
bursting or coming off, increase the typical failure rate to between
11 and 15 per cent.

The female condom

The female condom is a pre-lubricated, loose-fitting, disposable
polyurethane sheath measuring 17 cm by 8 cm.

It contains two flexible rings, one of which is attached and
remains outside the vagina. The smaller, inner ring sits loosely
inside the sheath in position beyond the pubic bone. The outer ring
may dangle between the legs initially, but lies flat against the female
during sex.

What puts most women off at first glance is the female condom's
size. In fact, this is an advantage as it gently lines the vagina,
allowing comfort and sensitivity during use.

Trials involving over 1,700 women using 30,000 female
condoms suggest they are as effective as other barrier methods of
contraception. When used carefully, failure rates may be as low as
2 per cent but can be as high as 15 per cent. The chance of a female
condom bursting is only 0.1 per cent compared to the male
condom's 8 to 12 per cent chance of breaking.

It is important that women who have just switched to using the
female condom should continue with their usual method of
contraception (e.g. Pill, male condom) until they are confident in its
use. Inadvertent slipping of the device, or the placing of the penis
between the female condom and the vaginal wall are more common
during the first few times of use.

The coil (IUCD – intra-uterine contraceptive device)

Modern coils are made from polyethylene and copper.

The coil is inserted into the womb using a technique which

carries a small risk of introducing an infection into the womb. Two monofilament threads hang down into the vagina to help removal and to allow checking that the device is still in place. Coils can be inserted immediately following childbirth or Caesarean section, but there is an increased risk of expulsion. They are usually fitted six weeks after delivery.

The recommended life span of many coils is from three to five years. Failure rates are 0.3 to 4 per cent.

Coils work in several ways to prevent pregnancy:

- Physical interference with implantation.
- Low-grade inflammation of the endometrium with infiltration of white pus cells (leucocytes), causing inflammation.
- Stimulation of hormone-like prostaglandin production.
- Copper ions are toxic to ova and spermatozoa.
- Interference with transportation of sperm and egg within the Fallopian tubes.

Removal of the coil is usually a simple matter of a doctor grasping the coil strings with a sterile instrument and gently pulling the coil out. In some cases, a coil can be difficult to remove and may need operative recovery under a general anaesthetic, although this is rare.

If the coil is to be removed, and you are not having another inserted, use condoms or another method of contraception for seven days before removal if you don't want to get pregnant.

Side effects

IUCDs may increase blood loss during menstruation, and as many as half of women fitted with a coil report heavier, more painful periods, which are the most common reason given for stopping using this method of contraception. The coil is also associated with an increased risk of ectopic pregnancy and an increased risk of pelvic inflammatory disease – especially during the first 20 days after insertion, presumably because insertion encourages the spread of infection into the female tract. As pelvic inflammatory disease can affect future fertility, an IUCD is not usually recommended for women who are at a high risk of sexually transmitted infection, or those with a previous history of ectopic pregnancy.

All these are good reasons for a woman wishing to start a family to have her coil removed at least three months before attempting conception.

The Mirena Intra-uterine System (IUS)

The intra-uterine system (IUS, or Mirena) is a hormonal method of contraception that delivers a progestogen hormone (levonorgestrel) directly into the uterus via a device similar to a coil. It consists of a plain, plastic T-frame whose vertical stem is surrounded by a hormone sleeve containing levonorgestrel which is slowly released into the uterine cavity.

The IUS acts as a contraceptive by:

- Changing cervical mucus to inhibit the passage of sperm.
- Suppressing the normal 'plumping up' of the womb lining (endometrium) so that a pregnancy cannot develop.
- Interfering with the development of ovarian follicles, although it does not completely suppress ovulation.

Researchers have failed to recover fertilised eggs from women using the IUS, and have concluded that it inhibits migration of sperm through the uterus and the Fallopian tubes. The endometrial changes it produces seem to prevent implantation rather than interrupting it and the IUS is therefore not considered to be an abortive method of contraception.

The IUS is as effective a method of contraception as female sterilisation (failure rate equivalent to fewer than two women in every 1,000 becoming pregnant per year), but is readily reversible. It is inserted into the uterine cavity by a trained GP or family planning doctor using a skilled procedure and a no-touch sterile technique.

It remains effective for up to five years before needing to be replaced, and releases a low dose of levonorgestrel locally through the delivery system to ensure low circulating hormone levels and minimal risk of side effects. Circulating levels of levonorgestrel hormone are much lower with the IUS than in women using oral contraception or the progestogen implant and are equivalent to taking just one to two progestogen-only 'mini' pills per week.

Another advantage of the IUS is that it is free from many of the side effects associated with normal copper IUCDs. It does not increase the risk of pelvic inflammatory disease (and may protect against it) and the hormone it contains reduces both the amount and duration of menstrual bleeding and can relieve heavy, painful periods. The risk of ectopic pregnancy is also lower than that for sexually active women not using contraception.

The most common side effect of the IUS is changes in menstrual bleeding patterns. When first fitted with the IUS, your first three periods may be longer than normal, and you may have some spotting between periods. A few women may bleed for many weeks, although this is not usually heavy. After this, your periods will become lighter and menstrual blood loss typically decreases by an average of 75 per cent. This is due to a local effect of levonorgestrel on the endometrium, which damps down the usual plumping up seen in response to the female hormone oestrogen during the first half of the menstrual cycle. For women with normally heavy periods, the reduced blood loss associated with Mirena will improve their symptoms and reduce the incidence of iron deficiency anaemia. It is therefore increasingly used as an alternative to hysterectomy in some women who also require contraception.

Around one in five women using the IUS find their menstrual flow eventually stops altogether by the end of one year, so they experience a total lack of periods (amenorrhoea). Amenorrhoea is not a major problem and many women welcome it. As it is a local effect of the progestogen hormone (levonorgestrel) on the womb, it is not associated with low circulating oestrogen levels (as may occur, for example, with longterm use of the depot progestogen contraceptive injection). A normal menstrual bleeding pattern will usually return within 30 days of removal of the IUS.

Other reported side effects include transient hormonal side effects at the start of treatment, which are uncommon and generally resolve after a few months. These side effects include headache, breast tenderness, skin problems and nausea. Some women experience lower abdominal pain, back pain and functional ovarian cysts. These cysts are a recognised side effect of progestogen-only contraceptives and usually disappear spontaneously without needing treatment.

Return to normal fertility occurs rapidly after removal of the IUS and the rates of conception in the first year after removal are similar to those seen in women using no contraception.

Removal is usually a simple matter of a doctor grasping the IUS strings with a sterile instrument and then gently pulling the system out. In some cases, an IUS can be difficult to remove and may need operative recovery under a general anaesthetic, although this is rare.

If the IUS is to be removed, and you are not having another inserted, use condoms or another method of contraception for seven days before removal if you don't want to get pregnant.

The combined oral contraceptive Pill

The combined oral contraceptive Pill (COCP) is one of the most reliable methods of contraception. It has a failure rate of less than 1 per cent as long as a woman remembers to take it every day. With poor compliance, failure rates are 7 per cent or higher.

The COCP contains two synthetic hormones, an oestrogen and a progestogen. It is taken every day for 21 days, then a seven-day Pill-free interval follows, during which contraceptive protection is still enjoyed.

The combined Pill works by:

- Inhibiting the secretion of follicle stimulating hormone (FSH) and luteinising hormone (LH) by the pituitary gland – without these, ovarian follicles cannot mature each month and ovulation stops.
- Thickening cervical mucus so sperm cannot easily swim through.
- Thinning the lining of the womb so if an egg does become fertilised it cannot implant or develop.
- Slowing transportation of sperm and eggs in the Fallopian tube.

It is now acceptable for women who don't smoke to use modern, low-dose COCPs right up until they reach the menopause. Women who smoke should stop using the COCP when they reach the age of 35 to minimise the risk of a blood clot (thrombo-embolism). The COCP may be started six weeks after childbirth or immediately following miscarriage or termination of pregnancy. It is not suitable for use whilst breast feeding.

Gastroenteritis can interfere with the absorption and contraceptive protection of the COCP. Women who suffer a bout of vomiting and/or diarrhoea should use additional methods of contraception (or abstention!) throughout the duration of the illness and for *seven* days after recovery.

Side effects

Possible side effects of the Pill include: nausea, headache, mood changes, changes in sex drive, intolerance to contact lenses, breast tenderness, weight gain, breakthrough bleeding, jaundice, blood clots, high blood pressure and, rarely, stroke.

Does taking the combined Pill affect future fertility?

In general, taking the Pill does not significantly reduce fertility as was initially feared.

Studies suggest that, among previously fertile women who stopped using the Pill, 90 per cent delivered a child within 30 months. This number is similar to that for women previously using the diaphragm or coil.

A delay of two to three months in the time taken to conceive was noted in these previously fertile women who had taken the Pill. This was thought to be a result of pre-conceptual advice not to conceive immediately after stopping the combined Pill.

However, a later study looking at older women aged 30 to 35 years who had *not* previously had a child suggested a more marked delay in conception. After stopping the Pill, 50 per cent of these older women took up to a year longer to conceive compared to those of the same age who had previously used a diaphragm. Conception rates were almost identical after 72 months, suggesting no permanent impairment to fertility.

Obviously these results are worrying. Few women aged 30 to 35 would want a delay of up to six years before conceiving once they had decided to start a family.

Does the combined Pill cause loss of periods after it is stopped?

Some women find they do not have a period for some months after they stop taking the Pill. In a study of 1,862 women in Sweden who stopped the combined Pill, it was found that:

- 3.3 per cent of women did not have a period until more than three months afterwards.
- 1.8 per cent of women did not have a period for over six months afterwards. This was most common in women under the age of 24 years.

Most specialists now think that any failure of periods to return after stopping the Pill is a casual observation, rather than a causal one. That is, a woman would have stopped having periods anyway, even if she was not taking the combined Pill. By taking the Pill, the regular monthly withdrawal bleed masked what would otherwise have shown up earlier as lack of a normal menstrual cycle.

Studies have shown that the different causes of lack of menstruation are the same between women who have recently taken the Pill and those who have not – and they occur with the same frequency. Also, the types of treatment given, the frequency with which these were used and the excellent outcomes in terms of successful conception rates were exactly the same.

Post-Pill fertility

In some women, fertility is at its greatest soon after stopping the oral contraceptive Pill. For this reason, the combined oral contraceptive Pill is sometimes prescribed to women about to undergo assisted fertility techniques such as artificial insemination to treat infertility.

In one study, researchers discovered by chance that successful pregnancy rates were twice as high in women given the combined Pill before in-vitro fertilisation, compared to those not taking the

Pill. In this study, the women had been given the Pill to ensure they were at the correct point in their menstrual cycles when specialists administered treatment.

It may be a shame to waste this period of hyper-fertility, especially for career women over the age of 30 trying for a first child. However, the delay in conception for 50 per cent of women aged between 30 and 35 years observed in the study previously quoted must be borne in mind.

What are the risks if a woman inadvertently takes the combined Pill during early pregnancy?

Women who accidentally conceive and continue to take the COCP during early pregnancy can be strongly reassured that the risk to their baby seems negligible.

Studies have shown that the rate of birth defects amongst babies born to mothers who accidentally took the Pill during early pregnancy are no higher than those expected in other women.

The Population Council estimate that only seven out of every 10,000 pregnancies exposed in this way result in foetal abnormality that might (or might not) be attributable to the Pill. The balance of research suggests a complete absence of risk.

Despite this apparent clean bill of health for the Pill, it remains important not to expose a foetus to any unnecessary drug, especially a hormonal one, during any stage of pregnancy. No one can be promised a completely normal baby as the risk of any important congenital abnormality is in the region of 2 per cent.

As well as suppressing fertility, the oral contraceptive Pill influences the blood levels of many vitamins and minerals. These are summarised in the table on page 33. Different brands and formulations of the Pill contain different synthetic hormones. Therefore, not all COCPs will cause all the effects shown in the table.

Vitamin A and the COCP

Circulating levels of vitamin A are increased immediately on starting the COCP and take three months to return to normal after stopping the Pill.

Although vitamin A is needed during pregnancy for normal foetal limb development, excess vitamin A causes birth abnormalities. For this reason, women who are pregnant, or contemplating pregnancy, are advised to avoid liver and liver products, which contain high levels of vitamin A.

As it takes three months for vitamin A levels to return to normal after stopping the Pill, it seems a sensible precaution to stop taking the Pill at least three months before trying to conceive unless the Pill's hyper-fertility effects are desired.

Vitamin B1 (thiamine) and the COCP

There is some evidence that the Pill affects the metabolism of vitamin B1 (thiamine), leading to lower blood levels and higher requirements.

In the pre-conceptual period, try to eat more foods rich in vitamin B1 (see page 64). If you have recently taken the Pill, a multi-supplement containing low-dose vitamin B1 may be beneficial.

Vitamin B2 (riboflavin) and the COCP

Taking the COCP for more than three years can result in vitamin deficiency. In the pre-conceptual period, eat more riboflavin-rich foods if you have recently taken the Pill (see page 65). A multi-vitamin supplement containing a low dose of vitamin B2 may be beneficial.

Vitamin B6 and the COCP

There is some controversy over whether vitamin B6 levels are decreased by the COCP. Studies suggesting that oral contraceptives cause vitamin B6 deficiency have used the metabolism of the essential amino acid tryptophan as a means of assessing vitamin B6 nutritional status. When other biochemical markers are used, it has been found that vitamin B6 nutritional status is not affected by oral contraceptive use.

Some authorities take the reduced blood levels at face value and suggest supplements of 50–100 mg of vitamin B6 per day. This is far too high and can cause symptoms of overdosage (see page 66).

Metabolic changes induced by the combined oral contraceptive Pill (COCP)

Substance	Blood level
Liver function	
• albumin	↓
• transaminase enzymes	↑
• amino acids	↓ and ↑
• blood sugar levels after eating starch	↑
• lipids (fats)	↑
• production of protective HDL-cholesterol	↓
Hormones	
• insulin	↑
• growth hormone	↑
• adrenal steroids	↑
• thyroid hormones	↑
• prolactin	↑
• luteinising hormone (LH)	↓
• follicle stimulating hormone (FSH)	↓
• natural oestrogen	↓
• natural progesterone	↓
Minerals	
• iron	↑
• copper	↑
• zinc	↓
Vitamins	
• vitamin A	↑
• vitamin B1 (thiamine)	↓
• vitamin B2 (riboflavin)	↓
• folate	↓
• vitamin B6	↓ ?
• vitamin B12	↓
• vitamin C	↓
• vitamin E	↓
• vitamin K	↑
• clotting factors	↑
• anti-clotting factors	↓ ↑
• blood viscosity (stickiness)	↑
• body water content	↑
• blood pressure	↑

Low dose supplements of only 5 mg of vitamin B6 per day are enough to overcome any possible deficiency associated with the COCP.

The Dietary Reference Value for vitamin B6 (1.2 mg per day) is exactly the same for non-pregnant and pregnant women – i.e. supplementation is not recommended.

If you have recently taken the oral contraceptive Pill, try increasing your intake of vitamin B6 rich foods (see page 82).

Folic acid (folate) and the COCP

Blood levels of folic acid are reduced by the COCP. Folic acid supplements are now strongly recommended for every woman who is contemplating pregnancy. These are especially important for women who become pregnant within three months of stopping the COCP. Supplements of 0.4 mg (400 micrograms) should be started at least one month before trying to conceive (see page 68).

Vitamin B12 and the COCP

The combined oral contraceptive Pill lowers blood levels of vitamin B12, but not enough to cause anaemia. Women who become pregnant within three months of stopping the oral contraceptive Pill are advised to take multi-vitamins that contain vitamin B12 as well as folate.

Vitamin C and the COCP

The COCP lowers blood levels of vitamin C. It is advisable for any woman (whether or not she has recently taken the COCP) to obtain at least 60 mg (European and US Dietary Reference Value) of vitamin C per day from her diet – and to supplement this with a 150 mg tablet as well. High blood levels of vitamin C are now proven to prevent many Western diseases (see pages 79 and 103).

Avoid mega-supplements of vitamin C, however. Doses of 1 g (1,000 mg) per day raise blood levels of the synthetic oestrogen hormones found in the COCP. In effect, this converts a low-dose Pill into a high-dose Pill and increases the risk of side effects.

Vitamin E and the COCP

The COCP lowers blood vitamin E levels by around 20 per cent. I would advise any woman, whether on the Pill or not, to ensure her diet is rich in vitamin E *and* to take a supplement of 50 mg vitamin E per day. Many studies have shown that high blood levels of vitamin E protect against diseases such as coronary heart disease and cancer. It is a safe supplement – even in doses 30 times greater than the recommended daily intake.

European Dietary recommendations for vitamin E are 10 mg per day, but 98 per cent of the population only obtain three-quarters of this amount. If you have recently been on the COCP, make sure you eat foods rich in this anti-oxidant vitamin (see page 81).

Iron and COCP

The combined oral contraceptive Pill usually causes light withdrawal bleeding. Less blood is shed through menstruation compared with women who are not taking the Pill. Haemoglobin, the pigment which colours blood red, is rich in iron. Therefore, by reducing blood loss, the Pill usually raises blood levels of iron beneficially.

Copper and the COCP

The COCP increases blood copper levels. It is possible that excessive copper levels are associated with high blood pressure (pre-eclampsia) during late pregnancy, and post-natal depression. This may be linked to its interference with zinc metabolism.

Zinc and the COCP

The COCP lowers blood zinc levels – possibly secondary to a rise in blood copper. Zinc is an important co-factor for over 100 enzymes, (substances which help biochemical reactions to occur in the body). It forms an integral part of the enzyme which switches on human genes in response to hormone triggers. By switching on a gene, this enzyme initiates the synthesis of the specific protein that gene codes for. Zinc is therefore vital in the development of the foetus.

Many cases of sub-fertility are thought to be linked to zinc deficiency. It may be beneficial for women who have recently taken the COCP to take a supplement containing 10 mg of zinc during pre-conceptual care, as well as eating zinc-rich foods (see page 99).

Should you stop the combined oral contraceptive Pill before trying to conceive?

Some specialists advise stopping the combined oral contraceptive Pill at least three months before trying to conceive. This is to allow the return of a regular hormonal cycle and to allow the various metabolic changes induced by the Pill (see table on page 33) to settle down.

Other specialists feel that, although this won't do any harm, there is no objective evidence to suggest that it is worth the effort. Becoming pregnant immediately after stopping the Pill has no significant adverse effects on the foetus. The only residual worry relates to alterations in maternal mineral and vitamin levels.

Opinions vary greatly on the use of the combined oral contraceptive Pill during the pre-conceptual care period. If you are in any doubt which is the best option for you, consult the specialist doctor who will care for your health throughout your future pregnancy and follow their advice.

On balance, it is best for a woman who is contemplating her first pregnancy or who had difficulty conceiving before to come off the COCP for at least three months prior to conceiving. It is best to stop at the end of a pack of Pills rather than stopping in the middle.

Women who have previously had difficulty conceiving should take the advice of their obstetrician on whether or not they should stop the Pill just before, or several months before, attempting to conceive.

A modified diet and/or nutritional supplements help to overcome the metabolic changes induced by the COCP.

Progestogen-only Pill

The progestogen-only Pill or mini-Pill lacks the additional oestrogen component of the combined oral contraceptive Pill. It is useful for women in whom oestrogens are contraindicated, for women over the age of 35 who smoke and for breast-feeding mothers.

The mini-Pill is an acceptable method of contraception during the pre-conceptual period if a couple are unable, or unwilling, to practise natural family planning techniques or to use a barrier method of contraception.

The mini-Pill does not necessarily inhibit ovulation. In around 60 per cent of cycles, eggs are still released. It works by:

- Thickening cervical mucus so sperm cannot swim through.
- Thinning the endometrium so if an egg is fertilised it cannot implant or develop.
- Decreasing the motility of sperm and eggs within the Fallopian tubes.

The progestogen-only Pill is usually started on the first day of menstrual bleeding. Contraceptive protection is then achieved within four hours. It is taken consecutively every day without a Pill-free break (even during menstruation) and must be taken within three hours of its due time to be effective. If delayed, cervical mucus starts to liquefy and contraceptive protection may be lost. Some users find a programmable alarm watch useful to remind them when their mini-Pill is due.

Most menstrual bleeds occurring while taking the mini-Pill are light and regular every 28 days. It is often prescribed immediately after childbirth as it does not interfere with breast feeding. Even if you decide not to use it during the pre-conceptual care period, you may wish to use it as soon as your baby is born.

The failure rate of the mini-Pill is very acceptable, ranging from 1 to 4 per cent. It seems to be less effective in women weighing more than 70 kg (11 stones).

Side effects

Possible unwanted side effects of the mini-Pill include:

- Menstrual irregularity or spotting.
- Total loss of periods (amenorrhoea). This is not harmful so long as pregnancy can be excluded. It implies that ovulation is inhibited. Some women are uneasy with absent periods and prefer to change to a different type of progestogen so menstruation can return.

- Ectopic pregnancy (fertilised egg implanting somewhere other than the womb, e.g. in a Fallopian tube).
- Functional luteal ovarian cysts (small cysts due to hormonal stimulation). These are of no real significance, but they may rupture and cause pain.

Injectable long-acting progestogen

The contraceptive injection is a slow-release store (depot) of a synthetic progestogen hormone (medroxyprogesterone acetate) which works by:

- Stopping ovulation in most cycles.
- Thickening cervical mucus so sperm cannot swim through so easily.
- Thinning the endometrial lining of the womb so if an egg is fertilised it cannot implant or develop.
- Decreasing motility of sperm and eggs within the Fallopian tubes.

The first injection (into your buttock or arm) is initially given during the first five days of a menstrual cycle (where day 1 is the first day of a period) to rule out pregnancy or within the first five weeks after childbirth. If you are breast feeding, however, the first injection is delayed until six weeks after delivery. After your first dose, the injection is repeated every 12 weeks as required (every 10 weeks in long-term users).

Always make sure you have your next injection on time, or there is a risk of unwanted pregnancy. If taking prescribed medicines to treat epilepsy or tuberculosis, always remind your doctor that you are using the contraceptive injection as these may affect the way it works and you may need to have your next injection a few weeks earlier than usual.

Although the injection works in the same way as the mini-Pill, it is more effective (failure rate usually less than 2 per cent) as it stops ovulation in most cycles. Minor side effects are common and menstrual irregularity is the rule, rather than the exception. Over half of long-term users experience absence of periods (amenorrhoea) by the end of their first year of use, and with some users amenorrhoea develops immediately. An internal examination and pregnancy test is then needed to exclude pregnancy. Long-term amenorrhoea associated with depot progestogen use is thought to increase the risk of bone demineralisation and osteoporosis – especially in smokers – although this is not yet proven. Some clinics measure oestrogen levels after a woman has used depot progestogen for five years and offer added oestrogen replacement if levels are low.

As the injection is a slow-release preparation, it does not stop acting immediately at three months when the injection is usually repeated, but may continue working for a while longer. Research suggests that women trying to conceive after stopping depot progestogen take at least four months longer to become pregnant compared with women stopping other methods of contraception. In some cases, fertility may take up to a year or longer to return so it is not a method for those wishing to conceive in the near future.

Progestogen implant

The progestogen implant (Implanon) consists of a single flexible rod, around the size of a matchstick, that is inserted beneath the skin on the inside of the upper arm under local anaesthetic. It is usually inserted during the first five days of the menstrual cycle and provides effective contraception for up to three years. In women who are very overweight it may not be as effective during its third year and may need earlier replacement. Implanon works by stopping ovulation, and also by making the cervical mucus thicker so sperm cannot swim through into the womb. It also has an effective on the womb lining. It is as effective as female sterilisation and is suitable for women wanting contraception for at least three years. Once Implanon is removed by a doctor or trained nurse, its effects are rapidly reversed and fertility is restored almost immediately. Most women ovulate within three months of its removal, and many ovulate during the first month.

Female sterilisation

Around 30 per cent of married, fertile women opt for sterilisation once they feel their family is complete. Unforeseen future circumstances result in from 1 to 10 per cent of these sterilised women requesting a reversal.

A pre-conceptual care programme is even more important for these women, not least because they are likely to be older than the average woman wishing to conceive.

Reversal of female sterilisation

Although female sterilisation should always be considered a permanent contraceptive option, in practice there is a 50 to 75 per cent chance of a successful reversal with subsequent pregnancy.

Reversal of female sterilisation is a major operation requiring open access to the pelvic organs through an abdominal scar, usually running along the bikini line. Where clips or rings were applied, these are removed and the extent of crush damage to the tubes assessed. Patency can be tested by flushing the tubes through with saline solutions.

If the tubes are blocked by scar tissue, or if they were originally ligated (cut and tied), tubal surgery is required. The blocked area is excised and the cut ends of the tubes carefully trimmed and joined (anastomosed). This is a skilful procedure requiring micro-surgical techniques.

After a female sterilisation reversal, there is a subsequent risk of ectopic pregnancy – where a fertilised egg implants in the Fallopian tube rather than in the womb.

Male sterilisation

Unfortunately, a growing number of women who wish to conceive are faced with the prospect of first having to wait for the reversal of their partner's vasectomy. This is particularly common where a man has experienced the break-up of a previous relationship and now wants to start a family with a new partner.

Reversal of vasectomy

A vasectomy should always be assumed permanent when a man first decides to undergo the procedure. In practice, reversals are frequently sought due to future, unforeseen circumstances.

Various methods are used but the technique is less important than the skill of the surgeon and the length of time between the vasectomy and its reversal.

Chances of success are greatest where a specialist uses microsurgical techniques and magnification from an operating microscope. This is because the vas channel being rejoined is only 0.25 to 33 mm in diameter. Often, the testicular end of the tube is dilated due to the pressure of semen building up, so skill is needed to join ends of different bore.

With the increasing passage of time, tissue changes (sperm granulomata) in each epididymis – a coiled tube at the upper pole of each testis – can interfere with the passage of sperm into the lower end of the vas deferens (the tube that carries the sperm from the testes). There is also an increased risk of the man making auto-antibodies against his own sperm, rendering them sluggish and interfering with his future fertility.

Various success rates are quoted for reversal of vasectomy. These vary from 30 to 70 per cent. One surgeon claims he expects an 80 to 90 per cent success rate in restoring sperm passage through the vas deferens and a 50 per cent chance that the partner will conceive within one year. If the vasectomy occurred more than ten years previously, the chances are less certain.

As a general rule, it is assumed that fertility can be successfully restored, with future fathering of a child, in two out of every five men (40 per cent) undergoing reversal.

Often men who have undergone a reversal of vasectomy have a lower sperm count than they achieved before the operation. Usually there is a significant improvement in sperm counts and the viability and motility of sperm over the following year.

It is important to wait for at least eighteen months for conception to occur. During this time, both the female and male partners should be actively following a pre-conceptual care programme to maximise their chances of a successful outcome.

If conception does not occur, all is not lost. The presence of viable sperm allows assisted fertility techniques, such as in-vitro (test tube) fertilisation, to be used. A new technique allows sperm to be aspirated from the epididymis using a fine needle. Semen may also be filtered to allow collection of healthy sperm when counts are low after a vasectomy reversal. Collected sperm can then be used for in-vitro fertilisation.

3

Pre-conceptual care
and a healthy diet

Pregnancy is a time when appetite is altered and nutritional needs are greatly changed. Advanced planning which introduces dietary and lifestyle changes before the challenge of pregnancy occurs is known to improve the chance of a healthy and successful outcome.

Why a healthy diet is important before conception

The most critical time of a baby's development is the first four weeks of gestation – often before the mother is even aware she is pregnant.

Recent studies suggest that the development of coronary heart disease, stroke or diabetes in later years is linked to growth failure in the first few weeks of life. If a baby is under-nourished at this critical time, it may become 'programmed' to develop high blood pressure, clotting disorders or abnormal glucose, insulin and cholesterol metabolism in middle age. This is not yet fully understood but may be caused by any of the following:

- Faulty development of the pancreas.
- Insufficient development of the placenta.
- The development of a larger than expected placenta.

One interesting study has shown that men born with the highest placental weight/birth weight ratio were at the greatest risk of developing hypertension (high blood pressure) in later life. This was thought to be directly related to maternal under-nutrition in early pregnancy.

Low birth weight

Babies born at optimum birth weights (3.5 to 4.5 kg) have the lowest risk of developmental disorders such as those of the central nervous system.

Unfortunately, around 47,000 babies with a low birth weight are born in England and Wales each year. These babies have a higher risk of physical or mental disability, with up to 8 per cent suffering severe conditions such as:

- Cerebral palsy.
- Mental retardation.
- Faulty development of the lungs.
- Blindness.
- Deafness.
- Epilepsy.

Studies show a significant relationship between the size of a baby at birth and the maternal diet at or around the time of conception. These first few weeks of gestation are a time of rapid division of cells. The central nervous system (brain and spinal cord) is often fully developed before the pregnancy is recognised.

Babies of teenage mothers are particularly at risk. Studies show their diets are low in iron, calcium, vitamin A and riboflavin, particularly if they're trying to lose weight with inappropriate slimming diets.

Low birth weight is also linked to smoking and excessive alcohol intake (see pages 154 and 161).

What is a healthy pre-conceptual diet?

Women preparing for pregnancy should follow a balanced, varied, whole food diet. Try to eat at least five portions of fruit or vegetables per day. This should average out at a daily intake of 400 g fruit and veg (not counting potatoes).

The healthiest diet is that found in Mediterranean countries and, in fact, a modified Mediterranean diet (without the alcohol) is ideal as a pre-conceptual and pregnancy healthy eating plan.

Try to avoid tinned and pre-packed convenience goods. Aim to eat only fresh produce and meals made from fresh ingredients. This will decrease your intake of salt and artificial additives and increase your intake of essential vitamins, minerals and fibre.

For optimum health you need the following elements in your diet.

Fresh fruit and vegetables

These provide minerals, vitamins and fibre which aid digestion and prevent constipation. Eat them raw or lightly steamed – without additional salt. Wash and where practical peel all fruit, salads and vegetables before eating. The potentially harmful effects of pesticides and fertilisers are not yet fully understood and therefore best avoided during the pre-conceptual period and during pregnancy itself. Aim for at least 400 g (around five portions) of fruit or vegetables per day – but the more the better.

Complex carbohydrates

These include wholewheat bread, brown rice, cereals, potatoes and wholewheat pasta. They are an important source of energy, vitamins and fibre. They are slowly digested and do not cause large fluctuations in blood sugar levels as simple carbohydrates (e.g. sugars) do. Aim to obtain at least half your daily calories in the form of unrefined complex carbohydrates. The pre-conceptual period is not a time when you should follow a low-carb (Atkins-style) diet as it is not known whether or not ketones are harmful to a developing baby.

Protein

Foods rich in protein include lean meat, fish, pulses, eggs, milk, cheese, cereals, nuts and seeds. Vegetarians can substitute fish and meat with pulses, grains, cereals, seeds and nuts (see page 105). US recommendations suggest that protein requirements increase to 60 g per day during pregnancy (non-pregnant dietary requirement is 50 g per day). UK Dietary Reference Values are slightly lower at 45 g per day non-pregnant and 51 g per day during pregnancy.

Most women in the Western world already obtain more than 60 g protein per day – e.g. the average daily intake among British adult females is 62 g. As this is only an average, 50 per cent of women will obtain less protein than this.

Try to eat at least 30 g (an ounce) of pulses, nuts or seeds per day as these are an important source of protein for vegetarians.

Essential fatty acids

Essential fatty acids (EFAs) belong to a group of oils known as long-chain polyunsaturated fatty acids (LCPs). While your body can make small amounts of the EFAs from other dietary fats, they are often in short supply – especially during pregnancy. You therefore need to get adequate amounts from your food, which is why they are labelled 'essential'. There are two main essential fatty acids:

- Linolenic acid (of which one type is gamma-linolenic acid, found in evening primrose oil).
- Linoleic acid.

Once in your body, these two EFAs act as building blocks to make cell membranes, sex hormones, and hormone-like chemicals (prostaglandins). EFAs can also be converted into two other types of LCPs that are especially important during pregnancy. These are:

- Arachidonic acid (AA) which you make from linoleic acid.
- Docosahexaenoic acid (DHA), which you make from linolenic acid.

If EFAs are in short supply – as they are in 8 out of 10 pregnant women – both you and your baby will be deficient in LCPs as well. In addition, your baby's metabolism is not mature enough to start performing these conversions on his own until at least four months after birth. He is therefore dependent on obtaining them from breast milk or enriched formulas, otherwise he will remain deficient during his early development when his visual acuity and brain cells desperately need them.

Essential fatty acids are needed for healthy cell membranes, nerves and hormone balance. They are especially important for the structure and development of your baby's eyes and brain.

Deficiency of EFAs is common during pregnancy

Research in many countries show that even in normal pregnancy, a mother's EFA status is marginal, with low EFA levels that tend to fall lower with each successive pregnancy. EFA deficiency is especially likely with multiple pregnancies.

If your diet is lacking in EFAs, your metabolism can make do with the next best fatty acids available, but this is not ideal. Every cell in your body – and that of your growing baby – is surrounded by a fatty envelope known as the cell membrane. When your diet is rich in EFAs, your cell membranes contain a higher percentage of LCPs and are flexible, healthy and youthful. If your diet is poor in EFAs, your cell membranes include more of other types of fat that tend to make them more rigid and prone to dryness, itching and premature ageing. The EFA content is important for the way receptors and communication channels fitted into the cell membrane work.

Developmental problems due to lack of LCPs

If EFAs are in short supply, they are replaced with less optimal long-chain fatty acids so that electrical transmission of signals between brain cells is impaired. Babies whose brains contain low levels of LCPs have significantly impaired brain development. It is now believed that a low-fat diet providing too few EFAs during pregnancy may be linked with an increased risk of the offspring developing dyslexia.

Dyslexia is a condition in which there is a considerable discrepancy between intellectual ability and written language skills. There is:

- An unexpected failure in learning to read and write.
- An unusual anatomical symmetry in language areas of the brain, which are more normally larger in the dominant cerebral hemisphere (the left side in right-handed individuals).
- Microscopic differences in the way cells are organised during development in the language areas of the brain.
- Difficulty in processing rapid changes in visual stimulation (e.g. flicker, motion).
- Impaired night vision (dark adaptation).
- Poor peripheral vision.
- Difficulty in processing rapid changes in the sounds involved in speech.

It is now thought that dyslexia is a brain development disorder linked with deficiency of certain essential fatty acids in the womb. This leads to mild abnormalities in the membranes of synapses in the foetal brain, which are less fluid than normal, and which transmit information more slowly. There is also evidence that lack of EFAs may lead to attention deficit hyperactivity disorder, autism and even schizophrenia, all of which are associated with dyslexia. Lack of dietary EFAs may not be the root cause of these conditions, but may trigger it in those predisposed to them through other genetic or environmental factors. It is also possible that the conditions are linked with poor ability to absorb EFAs from the gut, or problems with the way EFAs are handled once they reach the brain.

If your diet is lacking in EFAs, your baby will obtain a lot of the AA and DHA he needs from your body's richest store – your own brain. This may account for the slight shrinkage (2 to 3 per cent) in maternal brain size seen in some pregnant women, and cause the poor concentration, poor memory, forgetfulness and vagueness that many women experience during the last few months of pregnancy. By boosting your dietary intake of EFAs, AA and DHA throughout pregnancy, you can help to optimise development of your baby's brain and eyes.

Pregnancy is a time of rapid production of new cell membranes and itchy skin is common, especially towards the end of pregnancy.

Increasing your intake of EFAs will help make your skin feel softer and smoother within a few weeks. Anecdotal evidence also suggests that obtaining more EFAs during pregnancy may help to prevent stretch marks.

NB If you develop severe itching during pregnancy, you should always seek medical advice.

How to get EFAs from your diet

The levels of essential fatty acids found in your blood during pregnancy, and the concentrations found in breast milk during lactation, vary depending on how much of the essential fatty acids you obtain from your food. Oily fish (e.g. mackerel, herring, salmon, trout, sardines, pilchards) are the richest dietary source of EFAs and contain 10 to 100 times more DHA than non-marine food sources such as nuts, seeds, wholegrains and dark green, leafy vegetables.

- Docosahexaenoic acid is found in fish oils.
- Arachidonic acid is found in many foods, e.g. seafood, meat, dairy products, eggs.
- Linoleic acid alone is found in sunflower seeds, almonds, corn, sesame seeds, safflower oil and extra virgin olive oil.
- Linolenic acid alone is found in evening primrose oil, starflower (borage) seed oil and blackcurrant seed oil.
- Both linoleic and linolenic acids are found in rich quantities in walnuts, pumpkin seeds, soybeans, linseed oil, rapeseed oil and flax oil.

Unless you eat around 30 g of nuts or seeds per day and 300 g of oily fish per week, however, your diet is likely to be deficient in these vital building blocks. For the average person, this means increasing their fish intake by a factor of ten! Unfortunately, due to possible risk of pollutants, it is now recommended that you only eat fish twice a week, of which one portion is oily fish. If you want to eat more, make sure it is classed as organic.

Some research suggests the balance of EFAs in rapeseed oil may be better for brain development than those in olive, safflower or sunflower seed oils, so it may be worth switching to rapeseed oil for cooking.

Not everyone wants to make drastic changes to their diet, especially during pregnancy and not everyone likes eating fish. If this is the case, it is worth considering taking a supplement containing EFAs such as gamma-linolenic acid (e.g. evening primrose oil from which you can synthesise DHA) and one containing AA and DHA (e.g. fish oil supplements).

By improving your intake of EFAs through dietary changes, or by taking supplements, you can:

- Improve the development of your baby's eyes and brain.
- Improve your baby's visual acuity.
- Reduce your risk of pregnancy-associated high blood pressure (pre-eclampsia).
- Reduce your risk of a pre-term delivery.
- Reduce your risk of a low birth weight baby.
- Reduce fluid retention during pregnancy (oedema).
- Reduce your risk of poor concentration and scattiness towards the end of pregnancy.
- Reduce your risk of dry, itchy skin problems.
- Possibly reduce your risk of stretch marks.
- Possibly increase the intelligence of your baby through improved brain development.

How many calories do you need?

The Committee on Medical Aspects of Food Policy (COMA) report published in 1991 recommends the following intakes for women of reproductive age (see table opposite).

Calorie intakes for non-pregnant women are averages only. Half the population need fewer calories than those quoted and half need more, depending on factors such as height, current weight, metabolic rate, type of job and amount of exercise taken. The important point to note is that it is not necessary to eat for two during the first six months of pregnancy.

Overall, pregnant women need an extra 70,000 kcals during

pregnancy to account for storage in foetal and maternal tissues, the mother's increased metabolic rate and the extra energy she requires to move her heavier body around.

It is not necessary to eat these extra calories, however. The metabolism of pregnant women becomes more efficient and utilises all available energy rather than wasting excess as heat. Pregnant women also naturally cut down their level of activity and expend less energy in the form of exercise.

Estimated energy requirements for women (COMA)

Age	Kcal per day
11–14	1,845
15–18	2,110
19–50	1,940
Pregnancy	
0–6 months	as above, according to age
6–9 months	+ 200
Breast feeding	
0–1 month	+ 450
1–2 months	+ 530
2–3 months	+ 570
Where breast milk is the primary source of nourishment	
3–6 months	+ 570
6 months onwards	+ 550
Where breast milk is complementing active weaning	
3–6 months	+ 480
6 months onwards	+ 240

NB Women who are underweight before they conceive and women who do not decrease their activity levels may need more.

As above, there is now no longer a recommendation to increase calorie intake during the first six months of pregnancy. An extra 200 kcals per day are needed during the last three months of pregnancy and an extra 450 to 570 kcals while breast feeding.

It is important not to eat more than usual during the pre-conceptual care period or during early pregnancy. If you do, you may put on excess weight which can cause problems in later pregnancy and be difficult to shift afterwards (see page 109).

Modifying diet during the pre-conceptual care period

Often, the only adjustment needed for a healthy pre-conceptual diet is to cut down on foods of little nutritional value (e.g. biscuits, cakes, confectionery, pastries). This makes room for more valuable fibre, vitamin and mineral-rich fresh whole foods. Decrease your intake of:

- Refined sugar – ideally to zero.
- Salt – to less than 6 g per day. It lurks in tinned foods and biscuits, pastries, etc.
- Dietary fats (especially saturated). Eat no more than 30 per cent of daily calories as fat. Fat counters are available in newsagents to make calculation relatively simple.
- Highly processed foods jumping with additives.
- Red meat – three times per week or less is better than the more usual once or twice per day.
- Skin and visible fat from meat.
- Roast or fried foods, e.g. chips.
- Cakes, biscuits, crisps and pastries.
- Sweets and chocolates.
- Sugary, fizzy drinks.

Instead, eat more:

- Lean white meat, e.g. chicken.
- Fish – ideally twice a week, with one portion being oily fish (preferably organic).

- Wholemeal bread, wholewheat pasta, brown rice and plain potatoes – obtain at least half your daily energy from these sources.
- Fruit or vegetables – at least five portions per day.
- Vegetarian meals.
- Pulses, nuts or seeds every day – especially when cutting down on red meat. 30 g per day is ideal.
- Grilled, steamed, poached or casseroled food.
- Baked potatoes.
- Mineral water or fruit/herbal teas.

In general:

- Only eat when you are hungry.
- Eat little and often – e.g. six small meals spread throughout the day rather than three large meals at set times.
- Try not to eat late at night.
- Avoid alcohol.
- Exercise briskly (e.g. walking, cycling, swimming) for at least 20 minutes, three times a week.

A high-fibre diet

During the pre-conceptual care period, it's worth ensuring you follow a high-fibre diet. Roughage is essential – while it provides little of nutritional value, it aids the digestion and absorption of other foods.

Fibre encourages peristalsis (the muscular, wave-like motion which transports digested food through the intestines), helps regulate the bowels and absorbs water, toxins and bacteria. Recent evidence suggests that dietary fibre also absorbs fats and sugars in the bowel and can significantly lower our blood glucose and cholesterol levels too. This is because dietary fats and sugars are more slowly absorbed and also because more are excreted.

Fibre is an essential component of all plant cell structures – basically the parts which are indigestible. The main components are chemicals called cellulose, hemicellulose, lignin, pectins and gums. We lack the digestive enzymes necessary to break fibre down to release its energy values. Bacteria in our gut can break it down to produce acids and gases, however, in a process known as fermentation.

There are two main types of dietary fibre: soluble and insoluble. Soluble fibre is important in the stomach and upper intestines, where it slows down the processes of digestion and absorption. This ensures blood sugar and fat levels rise slowly rather than rapidly – and our metabolism can handle nutrient fluctuations more easily. Insoluble fibre is most important in the large bowel. It bulks up the faeces, absorbs excess water and keeps the bowels flowing smoothly and regularly.

All plant foods contain both soluble and insoluble fibre, though some sources are richer in one type than another. The following table gives some common examples of food rich in dietary fibre.

Sources of soluble and insoluble dietary fibre

Classification	Plant source	A few examples
Soluble	Oats	Porridge, muesli
	Barley	Pearl barley
	Rye	Bread, crispbread
	Fruit	Prunes, figs, apricots, tomatoes
	Vegetables	Carrots, potatoes, parsnips
	Pulses	Baked beans, kidney beans
Insoluble	Wheat	Wholemeal bread, cereals
	Maize	Sweetcorn, corn bread
	Rice	Brown rice
	Pasta	Wholemeal pasta, spinach pasta
	Fruit	Rhubarb, blackberries, strawberries
	Leaf vegetables	Cabbage, spinach, lettuce
	Pulses	Pease, broad beans, lentils

A high-fibre diet is important during pregnancy to help keep constipation and haemorrhoids at bay. It also controls absorption of nutrients from the upper gut.

If you are not used to a high-fibre diet, you must start to incorporate more fibre gradually to give your bowels time to adapt. By starting during the pre-conceptual care period, you will automatically be eating more healthily by the time you try to conceive.

The easiest way to increase the amount of fibre in our diet is to eat more unrefined complex carbohydrates in foods such as wholemeal bread, cereals, nuts, grains, root vegetables and fruits – all essential components of your healthy eating programme anyway.

Perhaps have muesli or porridge for breakfast, a wholemeal roll with lunch and a helping of beans as one of your five portions of vegetables or fruit per day. Aim for a daily intake of at least 25 to 30 g per day. As a rough idea:

Bowl of All-Bran	8 g fibre
Portion of wholemeal spaghetti	8 g fibre
3 tbsp cooked red kidney beans	6 g fibre
Bowl of bran muesli	5 g fibre
Jacket potato	5 g fibre
Portion of baked beans	5 g fibre
3 dried figs	5 g fibre
2 Shredded Wheat	4 g fibre
1 orange	3 g fibre
Portion of peas	3 g fibre
Portion of carrots	2 g fibre
1 average apple	2 g fibre
1 slice wholemeal bread	2 g fibre
Portion of brown rice	1 g fibre
1 slice white bread	< 1 g fibre

It is important to drink plenty of fluids (e.g. mineral water, fruit/herbal teas) for the fibre to absorb. Drink at least 2 to 3 litres of fluid per day.

Each gram of fibre you eat per day adds approximately 5 g to your daily weight of stool – so expect these to be bulkier. The additional weight comes from absorbed water and wastes plus bacteria that multiply from the energy they derive from fermenting your insoluble dietary fibre.

Common pre-conceptual care and pregnancy dietary questions answered

Should I avoid eating green potatoes?

It was commonly believed that eating green potatoes during pregnancy was harmful because they may contain a natural toxin called solanine. This was originally linked with spina bifida but that has now been disproved.

Can I drink coffee?

Recent evidence suggests that drinking three or more cups of coffee per day during pregnancy may increase the risk of miscarriage and drinking four or more cups of coffee per day may increase the risk of the baby suffering from sudden infant death syndrome (cot death). While this finding is still under investigation, some mothers may wish to limit the amount of caffeine-containing beverages (coffee, tea, cola) they drink during pregnancy.

Which cheeses are safe?

Cheese made from unpasteurised milk is likely to be contaminated with a bacterium called listeria (see page 147). Although it is relatively rare (one case per 30,000 pregnancies), it can cause problems during pregnancy. They are best avoided in the pre-conceptual period too. All hard Cheddar-type cheeses are safe, as are cottage cheese, soft processed cheese spreads and cream cheese.

Avoid
• Ripened soft cheeses, e.g. Brie, Camembert, Cambozola.
• Blue-veined cheeses, e.g. Stilton, Roquefort, blue Shropshire, blue Brie, Dolcelatte.

- Goat or sheep cheeses, e.g. feta, chèvre.
- Any unpasteurised soft and cream cheese.

Which milks are safe?

Blue, red and silver top cows' milk is safe to drink. Avoid the green-topped raw/unpasteurised cows' milk and all sheep and goats' milk (listeria and toxoplasmosis risk) unless it has been boiled immediately before drinking. Avoid soft whipped ice cream from ice cream machines.

Is yoghurt safe?

Yoghurts or fromage frais made from pasteurised cows' milk, including live, bio varieties, are safe. Avoid yoghurts or fromage frais made from sheep or goats' milk unless you know the milk was boiled first. Similarly, avoid unpasteurised (green top) cows' milk and any yoghurts made from it.

Are eggs dangerous?

Raw eggs and under-cooked poultry are linked with salmonella food poisoning. Everyone, including women who are or are intending to become pregnant, should avoid them. Make sure eggs are thoroughly cooked (set) before eating them – e.g. avoid runny omelettes. Avoid homemade mayonnaise made from raw egg yolk and homemade mousses made from raw, whipped egg white. Manufactured mayonnaise is made with pasteurised egg and is therefore safe – though watch the calories.

Is raw or undercooked meat dangerous?

Some raw meats are contaminated with a bacterium called toxoplasmosis (see page 148). This can have serious effects on the foetus if infections occur during pregnancy although it is rare (one case per 50,000 pregnancies). While preparing for pregnancy and throughout, avoid raw meat products (e.g. steak tartare, dried raw meats) and ensure that cooked meats are properly cooked. Also avoid reheated meat unless thoroughly recooked – it could also be contaminated with listeria or salmonella.

Is liver safe?

Women who are pregnant, or are contemplating pregnancy, should avoid liver and liver products such as pâté or cod liver oil. Liver contains high levels of vitamin A which can prove dangerous in pregnancy. Liver products also carry the risk of contamination with bacteria such as listeria.

Is shellfish safe?

It is best to avoid shellfish during the pre-conceptual care period and throughout pregnancy. Shellfish is a high-risk food for salmonella, listeria and other exotic contaminants such as poisonous plankton and heavy metals.

Are food cravings dangerous?

In one survey of pregnant women, 49 per cent admitted to having food fads. Many women find their taste sensations are altered during pregnancy. They may go off foods they liked before – or crave foods they previously avoided. As long as your food cravings don't prevent you from eating a varied balanced diet and don't make you put on excess weight, they are nothing to worry about. If you find you are craving unusual substances such as toothpaste, boot polish or coal, seek advice from your midwife or obstetrician. These cravings are more common than you would think – don't worry, you will be taken seriously.

4

Vitamins and pre-conceptual care

Vitamins are essential organic substances that have a specific bio-chemical function in the body. Most cannot be synthesised by humans (or not in sufficient quantity) and must therefore be obtained from the diet.

Vitamins are required in very small amounts and in many cases too much is as harmful as not enough. Pregnancy and the pre-conceptual care period are times when our vitamin needs are significantly increased. A varied, whole food diet is essential. In some cases, supplements are needed too. In most cases, adequate amounts of each nutrient can be obtained from the diet alone by increasing the amounts of vitamin-rich foods you eat.

To give an idea of how much of each vitamin your diet can provide, the following table shows the average intake of each vitamin for British women aged between 16 and 64 years. Against this is given the Recommended Nutrient Intake (RNI) of each during pregnancy. At present, the only supplement universally recommended during the pre-conceptual care period and in pregnancy is folic acid (folate) to reduce the incidence of neural tube defects in the foetus.

Some authorities also recommend vitamin B12 to further reduce the risk of neural tube defects or a multi-vitamin supplement to decrease the risk of congenital developmental defects in general.

The average vitamin intake of British adult females (16–64 years) plus Recommended Nutrient Intakes during pregnancy

Nutrient	Average dietary intake (UK adult reference nutrient intakes in brackets)	
	Females	*RNI (pregnancy)*
Vitamin A	1,058 mcg	(700 mcg)
Betacarotene	2.1 mg	(*)
Vitamin B1	1.2 mg	(0.9 mg)
Vitamin B2	1.6 mg	(1.4 mg)
Vitamin B3	28.5 mg	(13 mg)
Vitamin B6	1.6 mg	(1.2 mg)
Vitamin B12	5.2 mcg	(1.5 mcg)
Folate	213 mcg	(**)
Biotin	28.3 mcg	(***)
Vitamin C	62 mg	(60 mg)
Vitamin D	2.5 mcg	(****)
Vitamin E	7.2 mg	(10 mg)

(*) No RNI for betacarotene, but the National Cancer Institute suggests at least 6 mg per day.

(**) RNI of 200 mcg plus increased intake of folate-rich food plus a daily supplement of 400 mcg folate during pre-conceptual period until at least twelve weeks of pregnancy.

Women who have previously had a child with a neural tube defect need the RNI of 200 mcg plus increased intake of folate-rich foods plus 4 mg (4,000 mcg) of folate during the pre-conceptual care period until at least the twelfth week of pregnancy.

(***) No definite RNI, but biotin intakes between 10 and 200 mcg are thought to be safe and adequate. (US RDA = 300 mcg.)

(****) No RNI needed for people who receive exposure to sunlight. An RNI of 10 mcg is suggested for people confined indoors.

Sources: *The Dietary and Nutritional Survey of British Adults* (OPCS), HMSO Publication SS1241.

Dietary Reference Values for Food Energy and Nutrients for the UK, HMSO Publication RHSS 41.

At first glance, it would appear that most women are obtaining reference nutrient intakes of most vitamins except the important antioxidants, vitamin E and betacarotene. But an average is only an average – 50 per cent of women will be getting more than the averages shown and 50 per cent will be getting less. For example, although the average vitamin C intake is 62 mg per day, the observed intake range is wide, with some women only obtaining 14 mg per day – putting them at risk of scurvy – whilst others get as much as 161 mg per day from their diet.

It can be estimated that, using the future European guidelines, 60 per cent of British adults will not obtain recommended amounts of vitamin C (60 mg per day) from their diet.

The following overview of vitamins and minerals gives the daily amounts recommended for health in various countries and reviews research findings throughout the world.

Even in women who are trying to eat more healthily before pregnancy, intakes of many vitamins and minerals remains low. In one survey of 69 Dutch women, published in 2003, the 46 women planning a baby obtained more vitamins A, B1, B2, and calcium, selenium, magnesium and iron than those not planning a pregnancy. Even so, the percentage of women planning pregnancy with intakes below recommended levels was 74 per cent for iron, 59 per cent for selenium, 48 per cent for vitamin A and 91 per cent for copper. Dietary intakes of micro-nutrients in women planning a baby are far from ideal, and a multi-nutrient supplement is, in my view, essential.

In a study that looked at maternal use of vitamins in 538 women whose offspring developed a brain tumour, and compared these to 504 women whose offspring remained healthy, it was found that daily vitamin and mineral use in the month before pregnancy, and in each trimester, reduced the risk of the offspring developing a brain tumour (neuroblastoma) by 30 to 40 per cent. This study is consistent with findings for the protective effects of vitamins against other childhood cancers.

Multi-vitamins

Studies suggest that taking multi-vitamin supplements during the pre-conceptual care period can halve the rate of major congenital defects.

WHO scientists in Hungary gave either multi-vitamins (including folic acid) or trace elements to 4,000 pregnant women for at least a month before conception and a month afterwards. Women given multi-vitamins were half as likely to have babies with congenital malformations (14.7 per 1,000 births) compared to mothers given trace elements (28.3 per 1,000 births). The rate of *serious* congenital defects was also reduced by half.

Babies born with neural tube defects were not included in these statistics as these problems are already known to be reduced by folate supplements, so results were in fact more impressive than those quoted.

This study suggests that multi-vitamin supplements are a useful addition to a pre-conceptual care plan – especially for those who previously followed a nutrient-poor diet. Many teenagers fall into this category.

The dietary vitamin intake of Hungarian women, however, may differ significantly from that of women in the West. This may make them more prone to certain vitamin deficiencies and further research is needed to elucidate these findings.

As a general rule, sensible supplementation with a multi-vitamin preparation (avoiding megadoses) can only do good during pregnancy.

Individual vitamins, pre-conceptual care and pregnancy

Ensuring an adequate supply of vitamins and minerals just before and during your pregnancy is one of the most important things you can do for your growing child. The following pages look at a number of vitamins and minerals in some depth. It is important to obtain adequate supplies of all of them during pregnancy and foods rich in each particular nutrient are listed.

It is equally important not to exceed the safe doses of any dietary nutrient unless you are specifically advised to do so by your own doctor, e.g. if appropriate tests indicate a nutrient deficiency.

If in doubt over whether your diet is balanced or whether you need to take a nutrient supplement, always consult the doctor who will be caring for your health during the future pregnancy.

Vitamin A

Vitamin A is only found in animal products. As it is fat soluble, it is stored in the liver and most of us have enough to last at least one year.

Vitamin A is essential for reproduction, healthy moist eyes, vision, the integrity of cell membranes and for normal growth and development.

An extra 100 mcg of vitamin A per day is needed throughout pregnancy, raising the UK maternal RNI from 600 mcg to 700 mcg per day. The EC RDA for vitamin A is currently 800 mcg.

Most pregnant women in the Western world already have a vitamin A intake greater than this. The average pre-formed vitamin A intake of British women is 1,058 mcg per day, though observed intakes range from 134 mcg to 5,698 mcg. High intakes of vitamin A (3,000 mcg daily or more) during pregnancy have been associated with an increased risk of certain birth defects.

Foods rich in vitamin A include kidneys, eggs, milk, cheese, yoghurt, butter and oily fish. Margarine is also fortified with vitamin A by law. On average, women obtain 13 per cent of dietary pre-formed vitamin A from milk and milk products, 11 per cent from fat spreads and 6 per cent from cereal products. We get a massive 61 per cent from liver and liver products.

Too much vitamin A is poisonous, especially to the developing embryo, and is associated with congenital birth defects such as abnormalities of the kidneys and urogenital tracts. For this reason women who are, or might become, pregnant are advised not to take supplements containing high doses of vitamin A unless they are specifically advised to do so by their doctor.

Similarly, as a precautionary measure, it is recommended that women should also avoid eating liver or liver products (e.g. pâté) which have a high vitamin A content (and also pose a listeria risk, see page 147) during the pre-conceptual period and pregnancy.

Various vitamin A-like compounds (e.g. betacarotene) are found in vegetables. These are water soluble and cannot build up in the body to cause harm as they are flushed out through the kidneys.

Worldwide, vitamin A deficiency is a common and serious problem in underdeveloped countries. The safest way to ensure an adequate supply of vitamin A is to obtain plenty of the pro-vitamin betacarotene.

Betacarotene

Betacarotene is a powerful antioxidant, helping to overcome the damage to cells caused by free radicals (see page 101). When body stores of vitamin A are low, some molecules of betacarotene are split to yield two molecules of vitamin A. Zinc is essential for this reaction, so if zinc levels are low, there may be an associated deficiency of vitamin A. When vitamin A stores are high, beta-carotene stays as it is – and has its own important functions in protecting against disease.

Foods rich in betacarotene include dark green leafy vegetables (e.g. spinach, broccoli) and yellow/orange fruit (e.g. carrots, apricots, mangoes, red/yellow peppers and sweet potatoes).

On average, women get 70 per cent of dietary betacarotene from vegetables and 11 per cent from meat and meat products. Many women develop cravings for carrots during pregnancy. One woman chomped her way through a whole bed of young carrots, developing a yellow tinge to her skin due to a high blood level of carotenes (carotenemia). Pigmentation is not harmful and fades once carotene intake is reduced.

There is no evidence that betacarotene is harmful to the foetus at any dose level – even in women who were given up to 180 mg per day to treat a photosensitive skin disorder before pregnancy. Normal infants have also been born to women who were caro-tenemic during pregnancy itself.

Vitamin B1

Vitamin B1 – thiamine – is needed for the production of energy from carbohydrates and for the synthesis of some amino acids. It is essential for foetal growth. The amount we need is proportional to the amount of carbohydrate we eat. If we follow WHO guidelines and eat as much as 50 to 70 per cent of energy intake as complex carbohydrate, we need more but are also obtaining more from foods such as brown rice, wholemeal bread, etc.

The EC RDA for vitamin B is currently 1.4 mg per day. The average dietary intake of thiamine for British women is 1.2 mg per day, though observed dietary intakes range from 0.6 mg to 2.1 mg.

Worldwide, thiamine deficiency is common as body stores are usually only enough for one month. Those most at risk of thiamine deficiency are women on weight-loss diets and those drinking large amounts of coffee or tea, which destroy it.

Foods rich in vitamin B1 include wheatgerm, wholegrain products, oatmeal, yeast extract, brown rice, meat, seafood, pulses and nuts. On average, women get 37 per cent of their dietary thiamine from cereal products, 25 per cent from vegetables (mainly potatoes), 17 per cent from meats and 10 per cent from milk products.

Vitamin B2

Vitamin B2 – riboflavin – is also essential for smooth metabolic functioning and the production of energy – especially during pregnancy. We need a regular supply of vitamin B2 as it is water soluble and cannot be stored in large amounts.

The EC RDA for vitamin B2 is currently 1.6 mg daily. The observed average dietary intake of riboflavin for British women is 1.6 mg per day, though observed dietary intakes vary from 0.6 mg to 2.9 mg.

Foods rich in vitamin B2 include liver (avoid in the pre-conceptual period as well as in pregnancy), milk, cheese, yoghurt, yeast, eggs, wheat bran, green leafy vegetables, mushrooms, fruits, bread, cereals and meat. On average, women get 30 per cent of dietary riboflavin from milk and milk products (especially cheese), 22 per cent from cereals and 22 per cent from meat and meat products.

Vitamin B3

Vitamin B3 – niacin – plays another important role in the formation of metabolic enzymes and energy production.

The EC RDA for vitamin B3 is currently 18 mg daily. The observed average dietary intake of niacin for British women is 28.5 mg per day, but this varies from 13.7 mg to 46.6 mg.

Foods rich in vitamin B3 include lean meat, fish, poultry, yeast extract, peanuts, bran, beans, milk and wholegrains. On average, women get 32 per cent of dietary niacin from meat and meat products, 28 per cent from cereals, 10 per cent from vegetables and 10 per cent from milk and milk products.

Vitamin B5

Vitamin B5 – pantothenic acid – is one of the lesser B group vitamins. It is vital for many metabolic reactions involving carbohydrates, fats and proteins. Pantothenic acid is widely distributed and found in almost every food source.

The EC RDA for vitamin B5 is currently 6 mg daily. The observed average intake for British women is 4.5 mg per day, with intakes ranging from 4.4 mg to 7.7 mg. By eating more healthily during pregnancy, obtaining adequate supplies should not be a problem.

Vitamin B6

Vitamin B6 – pyridoxine – is needed for the proper functioning of over 60 enzymes and is involved in the synthesis of nucleic acid and proteins. It is especially important during rapid cell division, such as the formation of red blood cells and foetal development.

The EC RDA for vitamin B6 is currently 2 mg daily. The observed average intake for British women is 1.6 mg per day with intakes varying from 0.7 mg to 2.62 mg.

Many supplements are available that provide 50 mg to 500 mg vitamin B6 per tablet. Do not take high doses during the pre-conceptual care period.

Vitamin B12

Vitamin B12 – cobalamin – cooperates with folate during the synthesis of genetic material (DNA), a process that occurs continuously during foetal development. Deficiency of either vitamin leads to the formation of cells that are larger than they should be (megablastosis). Vitamin B12 also plays a role in the formation of healthy nerve sheaths (myelin).

Most experts now advise women who are pregnant, or contemplating pregnancy, to take vitamin B12 supplements as well as folic acid to help prevent neural tube defects in their offspring (see page 69). Recent research has shown that these defects are five times more common among babies whose mother had low blood levels of vitamin B12. The link found between low vitamin B12 levels and neural tube defects is independent of folate intakes.

Interestingly, maternal blood levels at which increased foetal risk occurs are higher than those usually associated with deficiency. As a result, current recommended daily allowances of vitamin B12 may need re-evaluation.

The EC RDA for vitamin B12 is currently 1 mcg daily. The observed average dietary intake of vitamin B12 for British women is 5.2 mcg per day, with the range varying from 1.3 mcg to 17.8 mcg.

Foods rich in vitamin B12 include fish, especially sardines, meat, eggs, milk and cheese. Liver is the richest source but is not recommended for women who are pregnant or planning to become pregnant (see page 63). Most adults who eat meat products obtain around 5 mcg vitamin B12 per day. No vegetables are known to consistently contain vitamin B12 – an important point for vegetarians, especially vegans (see page 105). Preparations of vitamin B12 that are made by bacterial fermentation and are therefore ethically acceptable to vegetarians are readily available.

Vitamin B12 deficiency is fairly common but is usually caused by malabsorption from the gut rather than dietary lack. This deficiency may be an undiagnosed cause of infertility as it can lead to ovulatory failure. In the United States, at least one such case was reported, involving a 32-year-old woman. She had unsuccessfully tried to conceive for five years. Tests showed she was moderately anaemic and she was given iron therapy and weekly injections of vitamin B12. Within one month she was pregnant.

Vitamin B12 deficiency can be masked by taking folate supplements, so B12 is usually given along with folic acid where clinically indicated.

The importance of folic acid (folate)

It's estimated that one in every twenty babies is born with a congenital malformation. Sadly, one in four of these is unlikely to
survive through infancy.

Most infants with birth defects are born to women with no
obvious risk factors.

One of the most exciting advances in the field of pre-conceptual
care was the discovery that folic acid supplements can prevent
neural tube defects. As these are a relatively common form of
unpredictable congenital malformation, this finding should significantly lower the number of babies born with such problems as
spina bifida, hydrocephalus (water on the brain) and anencephaly
(absent brain).

Other, less common, birth defects with which lack of folic acid
is associated are cleft palate, hare lip and abnormalities of the
limbs, heart, lungs, skeleton – and most other parts of the
developing embryo.

Folic acid (folate)

Is the only vitamin whose requirement more than doubles during
pregnancy. Its name comes from the Latin word *folia*, meaning leaf,
as it was first identified in spinach.

Folate is needed for a number of functions in the body:

• Formation of red blood cells.
• Metabolism of sugars and proteins.
• Formation of genetic material, DNA, during cell division.

Our body stores of folate are small and deficiency develops quickly.
In fact, folate deficiency is the most common vitamin deficiency in
industrialised countries.

Symptoms of folate deficiency in adults
• Weakness.
• Fatigue.
• Dizziness.

- Irritability.
- Depression.
- Cramps.
- Megaloblastic (large cell) anaemia.
- Diarrhoea.

Many commonly used drugs interfere with the way our body uses folate and can precipitate a deficiency. These include alcohol, some anti-epilepsy drugs (phenytoin, phenobarbitone, primidone), the diuretic triamterene, oral contraceptive Pills and the antibiotic trimethoprim (also present in co-trimoxazole).

In the average Western diet, we get most of our dietary folate from vegetables (35 per cent), bread and flour products (26 per cent), meat products (10 per cent), milk products (9 per cent) and fruit (6 per cent). The table on page 70 shows foods rich in this vital nutrient.

Although liver is a rich source of folic acid, women who intend to become pregnant are advised not to eat liver or liver products (see page 63).

As a rough guide, it is estimated that most people in the UK obtain around 0.244 mg (244 mcg) of folic acid per day.

Folate and neural tube defects

During early pregnancy, folate deficiency is associated with malformation of the embryonic neural tube. This is the early structure which will develop into the central nervous system (spinal cord and brain). These abnormalities are known as neural tube defects (see below).

Recent studies have shown that in women who have already had one child with a neural tube defect, folic acid supplements taken before and during the second pregnancy reduced the risk of a recurrence by 72 per cent. The evidence is so convincing that both the US and UK governments have issued guidelines recommending folic acid supplements for all women planning a pregnancy. Supplements are most effective when taken for three months prior to conception and in the first twelve weeks of pregnancy.

Good dietary sources of folate

Food	Mcg per typical serving
Fortified soft grain bread	105 mcg
Fortified cornflakes	100 mcg
Fortified branflakes	100 mcg
Brussels sprouts	100 mcg
Bovril	95 mcg (per cup)
Spinach	80 mcg
Oranges	50 mcg
Green beans	50 mcg
Cauliflower	45 mcg
Potatoes (old)	45 mcg
Yeast extract	40 mcg (used as a spread)
Branflakes (unfortified)	40 mcg
Wholemeal bread	40 mcg (two slices)
Potatoes (new)	40 mcg
Orange juice	40 mcg
Milk (whole/semi-skimmed)	35 mcg (one pint)
Broccoli	30 mcg
Peas	30 mcg
White bread	25 mcg (two slices)
Cabbage	25 mcg
Grapefruit	20 mcg
Lettuce	15 mcg
Tomatoes	15 mcg
Brown rice	15 mcg
Carrots	10 mcg
Sweetcorn	10 mcg
Spaghetti	9 mcg

NB 1 milligram (mg) = 1,000 micrograms (mcg)
Avoid prolonged boiling as this destroys much of the folate present in green leafy vegetables.

Advice in both the UK and USA is:

To prevent a first occurrence of neural tube defect

All women planning a pregnancy should consume additional folic acid before conceiving and during the first twelve weeks of pregnancy by:

- Eating more folate-rich foods including those fortified with folic acid (some breads and cereals).
- Taking a daily dietary supplement of 0.4 mg (400 mcg) of folic acid per day.
- Choosing foods which have been fortified with folic acid (including many breakfast cereals and some breads).

To prevent a recurrence of neural tube defect

Women who have previously had a child with a neural tube defect should take 4 mg of folic acid supplements (or 5 mg – available on prescription – if lower dose not available) daily. This should start before conception (I would suggest three months before) and continue until *at least* the twelfth week of pregnancy to help prevent a second occurrence.

Taking folate supplements throughout pregnancy

Some experts feel this advice does not go far enough. Mums-to-be may need folate supplements throughout their entire pregnancy. Biochemists believe this will reduce the number of babies born with a low birth weight – and also protect mothers against folate-deficiency anaemia.

Guidelines recommend that women take supplements of 0.2 mg of folate per day during the last six months of pregnancy, in addition to following a high-folate diet. Many women may prefer to continue taking their usual 0.4 mg supplement rather than dropping down to the half dose.

These recent findings concerning the protective effects of folic acid are so important, I cannot stress them enough.

To understand the significance of adequate folate supplies during pregnancy, it is useful to know how the central nervous system develops in humans.

Development of a normal neural tube

During the third week of an embryo's life, a thickening forms along the length of its back where the spine will eventually develop. The edges of this thickening start to grow upwards, forming a central

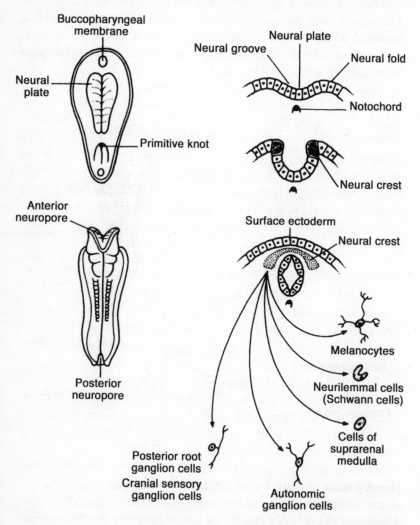

The formation of the neutral plate, neural groove and neural tube

groove. This neural groove continues to deepen and its walls fold over, until they meet above the groove.

Fusion starts halfway along the length of the neural groove and spreads upwards, towards the future head, and downwards towards the future coccyx. After three or four days, fusion is complete to form a long, hollow swelling called the neural tube. Cells grow over the surface of the tube so it becomes sunk into position, where it develops into the spinal cord. Three membranes, the meninges, develop like a sausage skin around the cord and these become filled with cerebro-spinal fluid.

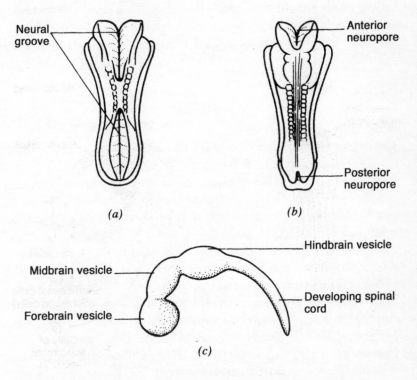

Development of neural tube: (a) neural groove at 22 days; (b) almost complete closure of the neural tube (later stage); (c) dilation of the cephalic end of the neural tube into forebrain, midbrain and hindbrain vesicles.

The head end of the neural tube dilates to form three hollow swellings which will develop into the complex human brain.

Groups of cells grow around the lower neural tube until they meet and fuse at the back. This encloses the developing spinal cord in a series of rings which will eventually become the protective, bony vertebrae.

The formation and development of the neural tube is a complex process. Healthy development seems to depend upon a rich supply of the vitamin folic acid (folate). This is essential for healthy cell division and the formation of new genetic material.

If folate is in short supply, cell division is hindered and complete fusion of the neural tube may not occur. This results in abnormalities of the central nervous system known as neural tube defects. Worldwide, there are an estimated 400,000 babies born with this problem every year.

Neural tube defects

Spina bifida

The most common type of neural tube defect is spina bifida. This affects around three babies out of every 10,000 births.

The spines and arches of one or more vertebrae fail to develop, usually with underlying abnormalities of the spinal cord and surrounding meningeal membranes. It can occur anywhere on the spine but is most common in the lower back. There are several distinct types of spina bifida, some more serious than others. The severity depends upon how much nerve tissue is exposed.

Spina bifida occulta is the most common and least serious form. The neural tube fuses correctly. The cells which grow around it in rings to produce the vertebrae develop properly throughout most of the length of the developing spinal cord. At the base, however, one or more rings of cells fail to meet around the back. The vertebral bones therefore develop almost like a horseshoe rather than a ring and the spinal column remains unprotected at the back. This defect is covered by muscles and cannot be seen from the surface.

Sometimes, the baby has a small dimple, a tuft of hair or a fatty

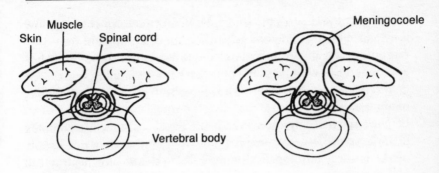

Spina bifida occulta

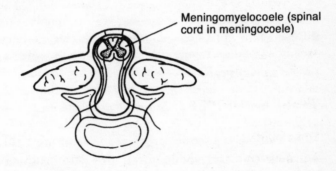

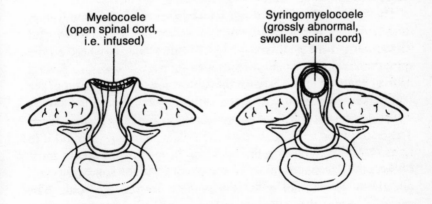

The different types of spina bifida

swelling at the base of the spine. Most cases are symptomless and only diagnosed by chance when the spine is X-rayed for other reasons. Occasionally, symptoms of leg weakness, cold or blue feet and difficulties with bladder control are noticed.

Meningocoele is a more serious version of spina bifida. The meningeal membranes surrounding the spinal cord bulge outwards between the defect in the vertebral arches forming a cystic swelling over the spine. Usually the spinal cord and nerves are intact and the defect is surgically repaired within the first few days after birth. Future development of the child depends on how much damage has occurred to the spinal cord.

Meningomyelocoele is similar to meningocoele except the normal spinal cord lies within the meningeal sac bulging through the vertebral defect. Surgical repair is more complex as the cord is stuck to the meningeal membranes and needs to be carefully freed and repositioned in its rightful place within the vertebral column. There is a greater chance of future problems such as leg weakness or paralysis.

Myelocoele is a serious problem and sadly most afflicted infants are stillborn. If the child is born alive, meningitis usually occurs within a few days.

This condition results from a failed fusion of the neural tube during the first few weeks of embryonic life. The spinal cord forms an oval, raw area at the base of the spine which discharges clear cerebro-spinal fluid on to the surface.

Encephalocoele is a rare disorder in which the upper part of the neural tube fails to fuse properly. Brain tissue bulges through the skull and severe mental handicap occurs.

Hydrocephalus

Hydrocephalus is an abnormal increase in the volume of cerebro-spinal fluid in the skull. When this problem occurs at the same time as spina bifida or meningocoele (see above) it is thought to be a result of the same underlying cause. When it occurs alone, it is not classified as a neural tube defect.

Hydrocephalus is caused by the abnormal development of the upper neural tube. Channels through which cerebro-spinal fluid usually flow and drain are either absent or abnormally narrowed. This allows fluid pressure to build up and the head swells.

Anencephaly

Anencephaly accounts for about half of all cases of neural tube defects. In this developmental disorder, most of the brain and the top of the skull fail to develop. This is due to a failure of the upper neural tube to fuse and develop so the top end remains open. Sadly, this condition is incompatible with life.

Risk of having a child with a neural tube defect

The number of babies born with a neural tube defect is now less than three per 10,000 births – compared to 40 per 10,000 births 30 years ago.

If a man or woman has had one previous child suffering from a neural tube defect, or if either parent is affected themself, the risk of having a baby with a neural tube defect is ten times higher than normal. If a man or woman has had two affected children, the risk of a third baby with a neural tube defect is 20 times higher.

It is reassuring to know that such a relatively simple precaution as taking regular folic acid supplements can help to prevent the above conditions recurring. Trials suggest that folic acid supplements can protect in 72 per cent of cases.

Taking folic acid

Awareness of the importance of taking folic acid is improving. A survey published in 1999 found that, overall, 45 per cent of pregnant women took folic acid *before* becoming pregnant. There has been a step-wise improvement from 1.8 per cent in 1993, 18.2 per cent in 1994, 27 per cent in 1995 and 30.6 per cent in 1997 suggesting that awareness campaigns have had a good effect. Even so, it is worrying that around half of women still do not use preconceptual folic acid supplements. This is most likely to occur in pregnancies that are unplanned. Unfortunately, moves to improve folic acid intakes in this group by fortifying flour with folic acid have been blocked in the UK. As a public health measure, the policy has been a great success with, for example, a 32 per cent fall in the incidence of spina bifida reported in the United States.

A recent analysis of four trials of folic acid supplementation involving 6,425 women has confirmed that taking folic acid around the time of conception reduced the incidence of neural tube defects by 62 per cent.

Over the last few years, several small studies have suggested that taking folic acid supplements may increase the likelihood of a mother conceiving twins. This was not thought to be because it increased the chance of multiple ovulation or of a fertilised egg dividing, but because folic acid is often in short supply during early pregnancy. Supplements that correct this deficiency were thought to increase the likelihood that, where a multiple pregnancy occurred, both foetuses would survive and progress to the stage where the twin pregnancy was recognised. However, a study published in the *Lancet* involving over 240,000 women in China showed that taking folic acid supplements to reduce the risk of a neural tube defect does not increase a woman's chance of giving birth to twins. Those taking folic acid daily were no more likely to give birth to twins than those who did not take folic acid supplements.

Precautions whilst taking folate supplements

There is no evidence that moderate supplementation with folic acid is harmful. There are two potential problems, however:

- Folic acid supplements may mask a vitamin B12 deficiency. Women who have recently been on the oral contraceptive Pill will need to ensure their diet contains foods rich in vitamin B12 – fish, especially sardines, meats, especially kidney and rabbit, eggs, milk and cheese. No vegetables are known to consistently contain vitamin B12 – an important point for vegetarians, especially vegans, who definitely need vitamin B12 supplements among others (see page 105).
- Some women on anticonvulsant drugs to control epilepsy may have a folic acid deficiency as their medications work by increasing folate metabolism. Relatively large supplements of folic acid (1 g per day) may antagonise the beneficial effects of

their drugs and increase the frequency of attacks. The level of folate supplementation you need should be carefully assessed with your GP or obstetrician.

Biotin

Biotin is a co-factor of several enzymes involved in the synthesis of fatty acids, purine nucleotides (which are building blocks for DNA) and in the metabolism of some amino acids (protein).

Biotin is widely distributed in food and is also synthesised by bacteria in our own gut. Deficiency is rare except in people who eat large amounts of raw egg white. This contains a protein called avidin which binds to biotin in the gut and prevents its absorption. Women practising pre-conceptual care will not usually be eating raw egg products, however, because of the risk of infection (see page 57). Avidin is denatured by cooking so it can no longer bind biotin.

Women following a poor diet who are also on long-term antibiotic treatment (which kills biotin-synthesising bacteria in the gut) may be at risk of deficiency, as are women following very low-calorie weight-loss diets. Severe biotin deficiency leads to hair loss and flaky dermatitis with anorexia, nausea and depression. Lack of biotin is also linked with severe cradle-cap in babies.

The EC RDA for biotin is 150 mcg daily. The average daily intake of biotin amongst British women is 28.3 mcg with intakes ranging from 9.8 mcg to 56.3 mcg per day.

Although apparently low, these intakes do not seem to cause signs of deficiency. They are assumed to be adequate to meet requirements because, on top of this, biotin is manufactured by gut bacteria and absorbed.

Foods rich in biotin include nuts, wholegrain foods, egg yolk, milk, sardines and vegetables.

Vitamin C

Vitamin C is essential for the synthesis of collagen – a major structural protein. It also acts as an antioxidant to mop up dangerous free radicals produced by the rapid metabolic reactions involved during the formation of the foetus (see page 101).

The EC RDA for vitamin C is currently 60 mg although this is widely thought to be too low. The average UK intake of vitamin C for British women is 62 mg per day. At first glance, this suggests that most of us are obtaining the European guidelines of 60 mg per day. But an average is only an average so 50 per cent will be getting more than 62 mg per day and 50 per cent are getting less. The observed average vitamin C intakes are wide, with some British women only obtaining 14 mg per day while others get as much as 161 mg per day. It is estimated that 60 per cent of adults may not be getting the recommended amounts (60 mg per day) of vitamin C from their diet.

Foods rich in vitamin C include blackcurrants, guavas, citrus fruits, mangoes, kiwi fruit, green peppers, strawberries, green sprouting vegetables (e.g. broccoli, sprouts, watercress) and potatoes. On average, 41 per cent of our intake comes from vegetables (13 per cent from potatoes) and 13 per cent from fruits and nuts.

Lack of vitamin C causes scurvy. Until recently, this was a relatively rare disease in the Western world but it is becoming more common – especially in teenage mothers who follow an inadequate diet. Many teenagers eat no fresh fruit or vegetables at all. In one recent case, a girl living on a diet of crisps, hamburgers, chocolate and cola developed bleeding gums, broken thread veins in her skin and dry fissured lips. She only obtained 8.5 mg of vitamin C per day. The minimum daily requirement to prevent scurvy is 10 mg. Interestingly, this girl was overweight and not anorexic. The other group of teenagers at high risk of developing scurvy are those with eating disorders (see page 119).

Vitamin D

Vitamin D is needed to help absorb dietary calcium in the gut. It stimulates synthesis of a calcium transport protein in the lining of our small intestine. Vitamin D is therefore essential for the growth and maintenance of bones and teeth.

We get most of our vitamin D from the action of short-wavelength, ultraviolet light on our skin. This synthesises vitamin

D from a cholesterol-like molecule in the skin. Our blood levels of vitamin D are naturally highest at the end of summer and lowest at the end of winter.

People living at high altitudes, those who cover up their skin in sunlight or who stay indoors all the time may have insufficient exposure to synthesise the required amounts of vitamin D. Dietary sources are then critical.

As most vitamin D is made by our skin in sunlight, the EC RDA for vitamin D is 5 mcg daily for younger adults. A reference nutrient intake of 10 mcg per day is recommended during pregnancy. The average British woman obtains 2.5 mcg of vitamin D per day from her diet. Intakes vary from 0.4 mcg to 6.9 mcg but we also synthesise it when exposed to sunlight.

Foods rich in vitamin D include oily fish (sardines, herring, mackerel, salmon, tuna), fortified margarine, eggs, whole milk and butter. On average, women obtain 28 per cent of dietary vitamin D from fat spreads, 26 per cent from cereal products and 20 per cent from oily fish.

Lack of vitamin D causes poor foetal bone development. An abnormally formed skull may lead to impaired brain development and future learning difficulties. Excess vitamin D is toxic, but this only occurs through too much oral intake and not through exposure to the sun, where synthesis is self-limiting.

Patients diagnosed as suffering from vitamin D toxicity were all taking more than 250 mcg of vitamin D per day. This leads to high blood levels of calcium with symptoms of thirst, anorexia, excess urine production and kidney stones.

Vitamin E

Vitamin E functions mainly as an antioxidant, mopping up dangerous free radicals (see page 101) that damage our cells. It is important in protecting our body fat stores and lipid cell membranes from damage and also protects vitamin A. It has been suggested that vitamin E can both help to prevent miscarriage and make labour easier through a strengthening effect on muscle fibre.

The EC RDA for vitamin E is 10 mg per day – 98 per cent of

Vitamins

Vitamin	Adult daily requirement	Why we need it	Where it's found
Vitamin A	1 mg	Growth, healthy eyes and skin. To fight infection.	Carrots; peppers; melon; liver; fish liver oil; watercress; apricots; dairy produce; green, leafy vegetables.
Thiamin (Vitamin B1)	1 mg	For metabolising carbohydrates, alcohol and some proteins.	Yeast extracts; pulses; nuts; rice; bran; flour; whole wheat; wheatgerm; sunflower seeds; meat.
Riboflavin (Vitamin B2)	1.5 mg	For metabolism of protein, fat and carbohydrate. For healthy tissues.	Liver; kidney; milk; yoghurt; cheese; yeast extract; eggs; wheat; mushrooms.
Niacin (Vitamin B3)	15–20 mg	For energy production. For a healthy skin.	Liver; kidney; meat; fish; yeast extract; peanuts; bran; pulses; whole wheat; coffee.
Pantothenic acid (Vitamin B5)	5 mg	Production of energy. Formation of antibodies. For a healthy nervous system.	Widely distributed in all foods.
Pyridoxine (Vitamin B6)	3 mg	For protein metabolism. Production of red blood cells.	Liver; wholegrain cereals; meat; fish; nuts; bananas; avocados; potatoes; beans.

Cobalamin (Vitamin B12)	3 mcg	Cell division. Red blood cell production. For a healthy nervous system.	Liver; kidney; eggs; cheese; milk; yeast extract; yoghurt; fish; meat.
Folic acid	200 mcg	For protein synthesis. Formation of blood. Metabolism of DNA and transmission of the genetic code.	Liver; kidney; dark green leafy vegetables; yeast extract; nuts; bran; oranges; eggs; some fish.
Biotin	100 mcg	Metabolism of food. Healthy skin.	Yeast extract; pulses; nuts; chocolate; wide distribution in food.
Vitamin C	30–60 mg	For healthy skin, teeth, bones and tissues. Aids iron absorption. For fighting disease and a healthy immune system.	Citrus fruits; dark green vegetables; potatoes; blackcurrants; strawberries; rosehip syrup.
Vitamin D	3 mcg	For the absorption of calcium and phosphate.	Fish liver oil; oily fish; eggs; milk; margarine; liver.
Vitamin E	10 mg	As an antioxidant to protect substances in the body from breaking down.	Vegetable oils; eggs; wheatgerm; nuts; wholemeal cereals; broccoli; avocados.
Vitamin K	100 mcg	Healthy clotting of blood.	Liver; dark green leafy vegetables.

NB Liver and liver products should be avoided during both the pre-conceptual care period and during pregnancy itself.

adults only obtain 8 mg of vitamin E per day, though intakes vary from 2.5 mg per day to 19.5 mg per day. The average British woman obtains 7.2 mg of vitamin E from her diet per day, with intakes varying from 2.5 mg to 15.2 mg.

Many experts now believe a daily intake of at least 40 mg to 50 mg of vitamin E is needed to provide adequate protection against free radical damage causing coronary heart disease. This means taking supplements, though they must be of natural source vitamin E (d-alphatocopherol), not synthetic (dl-alphatocopherol) which is less biologically active. Supplements of natural source vitamin E seem safe, even at higher doses of 3 g per day.

Foods rich in vitamin E include vegetable oils – of which wheatgerm oil is the richest – avocado pear, margarine, eggs, butter, wholemeal cereals, seeds, nuts, seafood (not shellfish) and broccoli.

Vitamin E content of various oils

Oil	Level of vitamin E (mg/100g)
Wheatgerm	136
Sunflower	49
Safflower	40
Palm	33
Rapeseed	22
Cod liver	20
Corn	17
Peanut	15
Olive	5

Vitamin E is easily transported across the placenta but premature infants are often born without adequate vitamin E reserves. As a result, their red blood cell membranes are unusually fragile, leading to a haemolytic anaemia and neonatal (newborn) jaundice.

Severe vitamin E deficiency causes foetal weakness, poor development of the heart, brain, lungs and kidneys. Developmental difficulties usually follow.

High doses of vitamin E are known to reduce the severity of eye damage (retrolental fibroplasia) caused by oxygen treatment of premature babies.

Dietary fat recommendations

Fat and calorie guides to help you estimate your fat intake can be bought in all good newsagents.

- Aim to eat no more than 30 per cent of total calories as fat.
- Aim to eat no less than 20 per cent of calories as fat.
- Saturated fat should make up less than 10 per cent of calories.
- Reduce pre-formed dietary cholesterol (found in eggs, fatty meats, dairy products) to less than 300 mg per day.
- Polyunsaturated fatty acids should make up 7 to 8 per cent of total calories and not exceed 10 per cent.

Painless ways to help achieve the above objectives

- Reduce the amount of red meat in your diet – e.g. to three portions per week or less.
- Switch to using olive oil, rich in mono-unsaturated fat. This helps to lower blood cholesterol levels and protects against heart disease.
- Increase your intake of oily fish (salmon, sardines, mackerel, herrings) to two portions totally around 300 g per week. These are high in essential fatty acids, help lower blood cholesterol levels and also protect the heart.
- Eat more vegetarian meals and have at least one vegetarian day per week.
- We need 5 g to 10 g linolenic acid per day. This is found in plant oils (e.g. groundnut, corn, soya bean, sunflower, olive oil) and chicken fat.
- Eat 30 g mixed nuts and seeds per day.

Vitamin K

Vitamin K is essential for the formation of blood clotting factors in the liver. Deficiency of vitamin K leads to prolonged bleeding.

Foods rich in vitamin K include green, leafy vegetables (e.g. broccoli, cabbage, lettuce). The other rich source, liver, is best avoided before and during pregnancy (see page 63).

Foetal levels of vitamin K are very low as placental transfer is limited. Vitamin K deficiency in the first week of life may cause bleeding in 1.7 per cent of neonates (classic early haemorrhagic disease of the newborn). Five out of every 100,000 children go on to have a major cerebral haemorrhage between the third and twelfth week of life (late haemorrhagic disease of the newborn). Therefore, babies are usually given vitamin K (by injection or by mouth) at birth. This prevents at least 40 children in the UK each year from having an intracranial haemorrhage. As babies who are breast fed are more likely to be vitamin K deficient than formula-fed infants, this preventative measure is especially important for them.

A controversial trial suggested a link between the administration of vitamin K by injection (but not by mouth) and subsequent doubled risk of developing childhood leukaemia before the age of ten. These results were not confirmed by a large Swedish study which reviewed data from 1.4 million births. They found that the risk of childhood cancer was no higher after intramuscular administration compared with the oral route.

The initial controversial study was repeated and again showed the link between vitamin K and childhood malignancy. The authors suggested this was enough evidence to only administer vitamin K by the oral route. Other doctors feel this is too radical a change and that it will put babies at risk of bleeding.

Vitamin K administration is definitely beneficial. Administration by injection virtually eliminates the risk of early or late haemolytic disease of the newborn. Oral vitamin K decreases the risk of late disease, but it is not clear by precisely how much. Infants may still be at risk of haemorrhage.

At present, it is up to healthcare professionals in each hospital to establish a locally agreed policy on how vitamin K is delivered. Parents anxious about children who have received intramuscular injection of vitamin K can be reassured that the risk is very small.

5

Minerals and trace elements

An adequate supply of minerals is just as important during the pre-conceptual care period and pregnancy as a sufficient intake of vitamins.

In most cases, recommended amounts of each nutrient can be obtained from your diet by increasing the amount of mineral-rich foods you eat. To give you an idea of how much of each mineral your diet provides, the following table shows the average intake for British women aged between 16 and 64 years. Against this is given the UK reference nutrient intake (RNI) of each mineral during pregnancy.

Average daily dietary intake

Nutrient	Females	(RNI pregnancy)
Iron	10.5 mg	(14.8 mg)
Calcium	726 mg	(700 mg)
Magnesium	237 mg	(270 mg)
Copper	1.23 mg	(1.2 mg)
Zinc	8.4 mg	(7 mg*)
Iodine	171 mcg	(140 mcg)

* New European guidelines for zinc recommend 15 mg per day.

Sources: *The Dietary and Nutritional Survey of British Adults* (OPCS), HMSO Publication SS1241.
Dietary Reference Values for Food Energy and Nutrients for the UK, HMSO Publication RHSS 41.

The average intakes of iron and magnesium are low, while intakes of calcium and copper are barely adequate. Again it's important to remember that the intakes quoted in the table are only averages. Some women will be getting more, whilst others are getting less. In fact, intakes of iron are skewed, with more than 50 per cent of women under the age of 50 years obtaining less than 9.8 mg per day (median intake).

All women who are planning to have a baby are well advised to re-evaluate their diet to ensure an adequate intake of all minerals. Low-dose mineral supplements are appropriate in many cases.

Mineral supplements

Some experts in nutrition believe that abnormal mineral intakes during pregnancy result in a wide variety of congenital disorders. One study looked at 20 stillbirths, 20 babies born with hydrocephalus and 20 cases of spina bifida. In each, they found a particular mineral imbalance:

- Hydrocephalus – high copper and high manganese levels.
- Stillbirth – high lead and high cadmium levels coupled with low zinc levels.
- Spina bifida – low zinc and low selenium levels.

The latter findings of low zinc levels in spina bifida may explain why women with adequate intakes of folic acid can still, rarely, have babies affected with a neural tube defect.

These specialists suggest that the mineral supplements on page 90 are taken during the pre-conceptual care period and during pregnancy itself.

If you are not sure whether your diet is adequate, or whether you should take mineral supplements during pre-conceptual care, consult the doctor who will be caring for your health during your future pregnancy. Medical opinions do vary on this.

Mineral	Additional requirements suggested for pregnancy
Zinc	an extra 10 mg per day
Copper	an extra 0.5 mg per day
Calcium	an extra 300 mg per day
Chromium III	an extra 100 mcg per day
Iron	an extra 10 mg per day
Magnesium	an extra 100 mg per day

Calcium

Calcium is needed during pregnancy for the growth and development of strong, healthy bones and teeth. It is also essential for muscle contraction, nerve conduction, blood coagulation, the production of energy and for the smooth functioning of the immune system. Adequate calcium intakes are important throughout life. Dietary deficiency at any stage significantly increases the risk of developing brittle bones (osteoporosis). Babies born to mothers with a poor calcium intake tend to have a low birth weight and slow development. The EC RDA for calcium is 800 mg per day.

Vitamin D is needed for absorption of calcium from the gut. Usually, only a small fraction of dietary calcium is taken up (typically less than 40 per cent), the remainder being lost in bowel motions. Interestingly, calcium absorption from the gut seems to be more efficient during pregnancy. This is secondary to a natural increase in blood levels of vitamin D – without any obvious increase in intake or increased exposure to the sun.

Foods rich in calcium include milk, yoghurt, cheese, green vegetables, oranges and bread. It is relatively easy to increase your calcium intake before pregnancy. The best way is to drink an extra pint of skimmed or semi-skimmed milk per day. This provides as much calcium as whole milk but without the additional saturated fat.

By law in the UK, white and brown flour (but not wholemeal) must be fortified with calcium. So, during the pre-conceptual care period, if your calcium intake is likely to be low (e.g. if you don't like milk or milk products), brown bread is the better choice. Regular exercise also protects against thinning bones.

Taking calcium supplements is not always beneficial as high levels of calcium in the gut interfere with iron uptake. Also, some supplements contain calcium salts which are not very soluble and pass through the gut unchanged.

A modified diet – starting before conception – is the best way to increase your calcium intake. Drink an additional pint of semi-skimmed milk per day – or take a low-dose supplement.

Calcium content of some foods

Food	Calcium content
Skimmed milk (600 ml)	720 mg
Semi-skimmed milk (600 ml)	720 mg
Whole milk (600 ml)	690 mg
Soya milk (600 ml)	78 mg
Whole milk yoghurt (150 ml)	300 mg
Low-fat yoghurt (150 ml)	285 mg
Cheddar cheese (30 g)	216 mg
Fromage frais (30 g)	27 mg
Cottage cheese (30 g)	22 mg
2 slices white bread	76 mg
2 slices brown bread	76 mg
2 slices wholemeal bread	41 mg
1 egg	25 mg

Source: *The Composition of Foods*, McCance & Widdowson's 5th edition.

Pregnancy-associated osteoporosis

Pregnancy-associated osteoporosis is becoming increasingly common. To feed the calcium hunger of developing foetal bones, calcium is leached from maternal bones and teeth when dietary intake is poor. This calcium drain from maternal bones is enough to cause weakening, and osteoporotic fractures are not uncommon. Hundreds of women are thought to suffer bone fractures during the last three months of pregnancy or in the early lactating period.

According to bone specialists, many cases of osteoporosis or of fracture are not picked up. Symptoms are dismissed as pregnancy-associated back pain or even as postnatal depression.

In one case where diagnosis was made, a new mother's bone mass was reduced to 50 per cent of the normal value for her age following delivery of her child.

Most women recover any lost bone mass spontaneously after childbirth so long as they have a high calcium intake, plenty of exercise and do not breast feed. Affected mothers are strongly advised not to breast feed as this is a further drain on calcium stores. Human breast milk contains 25 to 35 mg of calcium per 100 ml.

Chromium

Chromium is needed in trace amounts to form an organic complex called glucose tolerance factor (GTF). This contains vitamin B3 (niacin) and three amino acids as well as chromium. It is essential for the interaction between the hormone insulin and its cell wall receptors. Low levels of chromium are associated with poor glucose tolerance, as is seen in diabetes.

The optimum chromium intake is unknown but intakes are suggested of 50 mcg to 200 mcg per day for an adult. The average intake is below 50 mcg and it is thought that only 2 per cent is in an absorbable form. Deficiency is therefore common, especially among pregnant women. The importance of this is not yet fully understood.

Chromium deficiency and associated low levels of GTF may play a role in gestational (during pregnancy) diabetes. Some experts suggest obtaining an additional 100 mcg of chromium III per day during pregnancy, starting during the pre-conceptual care period.

The richest known source of natural GTF is brewer's yeast, whose GTF is ten times more active than that from any other food. Chromium-enriched yeast with an even higher content has now been bred. Other dietary sources of chromium include black pepper, thyme, wheatgerm, wholewheat bread, meat products and cheese.

Most refined carbohydrates have had their chromium content removed, another reason for eating unprocessed whole foods during your pre-conceptual care programme.

Interestingly, chromium levels are relatively high in newborn infants but decrease with age. This may reflect a dietary deficiency.

Copper

Copper is essential in very small amounts for healthy functioning of the liver, brain and muscles. Several metabolic enzymes contain copper, some of which are involved in brain metabolism. Others are essential for oxygen transportation and respiration. Copper is also essential for the production of melanin pigment and for collagen synthesis, maintaining healthy bones, cartilage, hair and skin.

Copper-containing enzymes are important antioxidants (see page 101) which either inhibit production of free radicals or mop them up once they are formed.

Adult women need around 1.2 mg copper per day to prevent copper deficiency. No increment is specifically suggested during pregnancy, although up to an additional 0.5 mg per day is recommended during lactation. Some experts feel this additional 0.5 mg is needed during pregnancy as well. The desirable copper intake to promote optimal health is not yet agreed. Some specialists advocate obtaining 1.5 mg to 3 mg of copper per day.

The observed average intake of copper among British women is 1.23 mg per day although only around 30 per cent of this is absorbed. Absorption is decreased by the presence of raw meat or excessive vitamin C, zinc and calcium in the intestines.

Foods rich in copper include crustaceans, nuts, dried stone fruits, dried peas or beans and green vegetables. Plant copper levels vary depending on the copper content of the soil in which they were grown.

Copper is toxic in excess and as gross deficiency is relatively rare, only diet sources or low-dose supplements (e.g. 0.5 mg per day) are recommended.

NB Copper and zinc antagonise one another and symptoms of copper deficiency (anaemia, low white blood cell count, sub-fertility, elevated blood cholesterol, thinning bones) have been seen in patients taking zinc supplements in large amounts for over a year.

Levels of zinc supplementation in the region of 10 mg to 15 mg per day are unlikely to produce severe copper deficiency. In general, we need a zinc to copper intake ratio of 10 zinc:1 copper.

The oral contraceptive Pill can cause blood copper levels to increase and zinc levels to decrease (see page 35).

Iodine

Iodine is essential for the synthesis of thyroid hormones. In the foetus, adequate supplies are also needed for development of the central nervous system during at least the first three months' gestation.

Iodine requirements rise by 25 mcg during pregnancy, from 150 mcg to 175 mcg per day (USA recommendations). This increased need is taken for granted in Britain as iodine deficiency is now rare since the introduction of iodised salt.

Foods rich in iodine include marine fish, seafood (e.g. shrimps, lobster), seaweeds and iodised salt. In the UK, cows' milk is also a good source as a result of the iodisation of cattle feed.

In some areas of the world, including parts of Europe, iodine deficiency leads to endemic goitre (grossly enlarged thyroid gland). In parts of central Brazil and the Himalayas, goitres affect more than 90 per cent of the population.

Because selenium also plays a role in the metabolism of thyroid hormones, the effects of iodine deficiency are exacerbated by low selenium intakes. This was reported in New Zealand, before iodine supplementation of food and agricultural enrichment with selenium occurred.

In underdeveloped countries where iodine deficiency occurs, expectant mothers are at risk of giving birth to hypothyroid babies (cretinism) in which physical and mental retardation occurs. Pre-conceptual (or early pregnancy) injection with iodised oil can prevent this.

Iron

Iron is an essential component of haemoglobin, the red blood cell protein which carries oxygen from the lungs to the tissues and carbon dioxide back to the lungs for excretion. Iron is also needed during the combustion of food with oxygen to produce energy and water.

During pregnancy, iron requirements increase as maternal red blood cell mass increases by 30 per cent. The developing foetus is developing its own blood stores too. Overall, an extra 550 mg of iron is needed throughout pregnancy – 300 mg for the foetus, 50 mg for the placenta and 200 mg to account for blood lost during childbirth.

After three months of pregnancy, the mother's red blood cell mass increases by an amount equal to another 500 mg of iron, which is usually borrowed from internal stores rather than requiring an additional intake. Against these extra needs of pregnancy, there is a saving of around 200 mg iron from the lack of menstruation and from improved uptake of iron from the gut.

Worldwide, iron deficiency is probably the commonest nutritional disease, with most cases going unrecognised.

The EC RDA for iron is 14 mg per day. It is generally believed that women of childbearing age have sufficient iron stores to cope with pregnancy and, in fact, no increment is suggested during pregnancy unless a woman has previously had heavy periods (putting her at risk of iron deficiency anaemia).

The observed iron intake for British women is only 10.5 mg per day, which is 30 per cent lower than recommended. As many as 50 per cent of women obtain less than 9.7 mg per day. This suggests that the majority of women should consider changing their diet during the pre-conceptual care period and throughout pregnancy. Only take iron supplements if recommended by your doctor, however.

Previously, there was a universal policy for prescribing iron supplements to all pregnant women. This is now less common as cheap supplements can cause constipation or indigestion. Iron is no longer given routinely except to women with a history of anaemia, heavy periods, a poor diet, multiple pregnancies or repeated pregnancies. In some cases, supplements of 30 mg to 60 mg of iron per day are prescribed under medical supervision.

Blood tests are taken at around twelve weeks' gestation and repeated at 28 to 30 weeks of pregnancy. If these show a low haemoglobin level, iron supplements are prescribed.

Foods providing iron include red meat, poultry, fish, nuts, wholemeal bread, cocoa, egg yolk, green vegetables and parsley. Over-boiling vegetables decreases their iron availability by up to 20 per cent.

Vitamin C increases the absorption of iron while calcium and tannin-containing drinks (e.g. tea) decrease it. Iron supplements given alone can decrease the absorption of zinc and other essential minerals (e.g. manganese, chromium and selenium) so some specialists advise iron is given in combination with these.

Magnesium

Magnesium is the third commonest mineral inside body cells after potassium and phosphorus. It is needed for every major biological process from the synthesis of protein and DNA to glucose metabolism, energy production and enzyme function. It is essential for healthy tissues, including heart muscle and nerve cells. The EC RDA for magnesium is 300 mg.

Magnesium deficiency is common. The observed average daily intake of magnesium among British women is 237 mg per day, which is significantly below the recommended level. Some nutritionists recommend that supplements of 100 mg magnesium per day are taken during the pre-conceptual period and throughout pregnancy. Magnesium gluconate seems less likely to cause diarrhoea than other supplementary compounds.

Foods rich in magnesium include nuts, seafood, seaweed, soya beans, meat, eggs, milk, dairy products and wholegrains. Magnesium is found in chlorophyll, the green pigment in plants, so green leafy vegetables are a rich source of magnesium – the greener the better.

Drinking water from hard-water areas is another important source of dietary magnesium. On average, we obtain 33 per cent of our magnesium intake from cereals and 18 per cent from green vegetables.

A diet high in refined and processed food will be deficient in magnesium as well as other important minerals, vitamins and fibre. Magnesium deficiency is associated with poor appetite, tiredness, insomnia, constipation, muscular spasms, twitches and cramps.

Lack of magnesium is exacerbated by pregnancy and some researchers believe deficiency contributes to miscarriage, premature delivery and also painful contractions during childbirth.

Magnesium has also been used as a treatment for high blood pressure during pregnancy, presumably to overcome spasm in the muscle of arterial walls. It has been suggested by some scientists that magnesium may protect against coronary heart disease in the same way.

Manganese

Manganese is an important antioxidant which helps to protect us from free radical attack (see page 101). Its other roles are not fully understood, though it may be important in the synthesis of blood clotting factors and cholesterol. It is also involved in brain physiology, particularly in the synthesis of the neuro-transmitter dopamine. Lack of manganese is associated with reduced fertility, poor foetal growth, birth defect and stillbirth in animals.

On average, we lose around 4 mg manganese per day in our waste products, which needs replacing. The optimal intake of manganese is unknown. A daily intake of 2 to 5 mg is believed to be adequate, while up to 10 mg per day is safe. The observed average intake among British women is 5.5 mg for pregnant women, but only 3.3 mg among non-pregnant women.

Foods rich in manganese include wholegrains, nuts, fruits, seeds, yeast, eggs and leafy, green vegetables or herbs – depending on the manganese content and acidity of the soil in which they were grown. Other sources include meat, seafood and milk. Tea is an exceptionally rich source – it is estimated that in

Britain, half our daily intake of manganese comes from drinking tea!

Manganese is one of the least toxic minerals, as when excess is consumed in the diet, absorption is very low while excretion (via the bile and kidneys) is high.

Selenium

Selenium is a powerful antioxidant that helps to protect us against free radical attack (see page 101). It is essential for cell growth and fighting infection but is only required in minute quantities. Selenium performs many of its functions in association with vitamin E, another important antioxidant.

The UK female reference nutrient intake for selenium is 60 mcg per day. No increment is suggested during pregnancy, although an additional 15 mcg per day is suggested during lactation.

Excess selenium can be toxic. An upper safe limit of 450 mcg per day has been suggested for adult males. Women should ensure their intake is below this level. If supplements are used, they should contain between 50 and 200 mcg selenium and no more unless prescribed under medical supervision. Additional vitamin E should be taken too.

Interestingly, inorganic selenium (but not organic) should be taken at a different time to vitamin C, for the latter impairs inorganic selenium absorption.

Foods rich in selenium include broccoli, mushrooms, cabbage, radishes, onions, garlic, celery, fish, wholegrains, wheatgerm, nuts and yeast. A selenium-enriched strain of organic yeast is now also available.

The observed average intake of selenium in the UK is 65 mcg per day, with 50 per cent obtained from cereals. Meat and fish provide most of the rest.

Lack of selenium in the soil does not affect plant growth, but can cause a muscle-wasting disease in grazing animals as a result of deficiency. Soil levels are so low in parts of the US, New Zealand and Finland that selenium is added to fertilisers to increase the population intake. In China, intakes of selenium are less than 12 mcg per day, which is associated with an endemic weakness of heart muscle (Keshan disease) that is responsive to selenium supplementation. Average selenium intakes among the New Zealand population are 15 mcg to 40 mcg per day, although no selenium-responsive disease has so far been identified.

Selenium may be important in preventing cot death. In the USA, a quarter of babies who died from sudden infant death syndrome were found to be deficient in selenium and/or vitamin E. Most of these had been bottle fed rather than breast fed.

Zinc

Zinc is an important co-factor for over a hundred different enzymes. It forms an integral part of an enzyme which switches on human genes in response to a hormone trigger. By switching on a gene, it initiates synthesis of the specific protein that gene codes for. Zinc is therefore vital in the development of the foetus. Recent studies also suggest that zinc is essential for functioning of the immune system and to prevent degeneration of vision with increasing age.

The EC RDA for zinc is 15 mg per day. The observed average zinc intake amongst British women is only 8.4 mg per day – 30 per cent less than the new European recommendation. Studies show that most pregnant women obtain less dietary zinc than the EC RDA and supplements seem advisable.

Foods rich in zinc include oatmeal, wholegrain products, yeast, seafoods, meat, nuts, milk, eggs and cheese. Moderate amounts of zinc are found in chicken and vegetables. In general, animal meat is a better source of bio-available (absorbable) zinc than vegetables.

Maternal blood zinc levels fall by around 30 per cent during pregnancy. This is not preventable by zinc supplementation and may represent the normal pregnancy effect of blood dilation. Zinc levels in foetal blood are usually double those of the mother's blood.

This maternal effect may be secondary to changing hormone levels. Zinc levels also fall while taking the oral contraceptive Pill (see page 35) and some researchers believe that lowered blood levels of zinc in pregnancy may not represent a true deficiency. However, zinc levels of maternal white blood cells are significantly lower in mothers who have small birth weight babies, so further research is needed.

Recent research has shown that babies given low-dose zinc supplements after birth grew significantly faster than babies fed normally. The difference was most noticeable in boys. The researcher concluded that infants breast fed for more than four months may show a slower rate of growth due to zinc deficiency. Other studies have suggested that zinc increases the size of the penis and testes in growing boys.

Zinc deficiency occurs mainly in people in hot countries whose diet is based on unleavened wholemeal bread. Wheat flour contains little zinc and that which is present is bound to a plant substance, phytate. In addition, sweat has a high zinc content, so the climate contributes to low zinc levels in the body.

Zinc plays a major role in the sensitivity of tissues to sex hormones and this deficiency mainly manifests itself as delayed puberty – males aged eighteen to twenty can still be prepubertal. Less severe zinc deficiencies cause poor wound healing and depressed sensations of taste and smell.

If your zinc levels are low, taking supplements of 15 mg zinc per day will cause a rapid improvement. If you find this level in zinc intake causes gastrointestinal symptoms such as nausea, drop down to taking supplements of 10 mg per day.

It's worth bearing in mind that soya products and foods rich in iron reduce the absorption of zinc from the gut. They are best avoided within two hours of taking your supplements.

Other minerals

Phosphorus and potassium are so widely available from our diet that we don't need to worry about deficiency. Other trace elements such as cobalt, nickel, molybdenum, etc. are not mentioned here as ample amounts for health are obtained from a normal diet rich in pulses, wholegrains and vegetables.

6

Antioxidants and free radicals

Several protective substances in our diet help to prevent oxidating chemical reactions from damaging our cells (see below). These substances are known collectively as antioxidants and include the so-called super vitamins A, C, E and carotenoids plus the minerals selenium and zinc.

Antioxidants exert their protective effect by mopping up dangerous free radicals.

What are free radicals?

As in real life, a free radical is a highly unstable entity that races round picking fights and causing damage.

The chemical version consists of highly unstable molecular fragments which carry a negative electrical charge. They race around, banging into other molecules in an attempt to neutralise themselves – either by stealing a positive charge or off-loading their own negative one. This process is known as *oxidation*.

Body proteins, fats, cell membranes and even our genetic material (DNA) are constantly under attack. It is estimated that every cell in our body is subjected to 10,000 free radical oxidations per day. Our main defence against these attacks is antioxidants. Antioxidants mop up unstable free radicals, neutralising their negative charge before they can do any harm.

What causes free radicals?

Free radicals are generated in a number of ways. These include:

- Normal metabolic reactions.
- Cigarette smoke.
- Exhaust fumes.
- X-ray irradiation.
- UVA sunlight rays.
- Alcohol.
- Drugs – especially antibiotics.

What harm do free radicals do?

Free radicals damage cellular molecules through oxidation. Oxidation of cell lipid membranes and fat stores is associated with premature wrinkling of the skin. Oxidation of cholesterol hastens furring and hardening of the arteries leading to coronary heart disease. If our genetic material – the DNA template in each cell nucleus – is oxidised, errors can occur when chromosomes are duplicated during cell division. This leads to mutations which affect future cell division. In extreme cases, malignant cells (cancers) are triggered.

If DNA in the sperm or eggs is damaged by oxidation, several undesirable outcomes are possible:

- The damaged sperm or egg may not be capable of fertilisation.
- Damaged genes may be passed on to the developing foetus if fertilisation is successful.
- The foetus may develop a congenital birth defect.
- The foetus may grow slowly and be small for dates.
- The offspring may develop a childhood cancer.
- The offspring may pass on genetic defects to future generations with unpredictable consequences.

It is therefore worth ensuring an adequate supply of antioxidant vitamins and minerals during the pre-conceptual period. This is especially important for men, in whom it takes around 100 days to make a sperm. The millions of sperm that are ejaculated when conception is attempted can therefore be maximally protected (see page 185).

In women, each egg cell is present since birth. Two important further egg cell divisions occur at the time of ovulation and at fertilisation, so although long-term protection may not have been provided, it is advisable to ensure adequate levels of antioxidants now. Antioxidants obtained during the pre-conceptual care period will protect these two important final egg divisions.

Similarly, foetal development is a time of rapid cell division with billions of chromosomal replications occurring. Antioxidants are therefore important throughout pregnancy too.

Researchers have analysed blood levels of antioxidants in large numbers of people and followed them up to see who developed coronary heart disease and cancer. Those with the least risk of these diseases are those with the highest circulating levels of protective antioxidants. When calculating the daily intake of antioxidant vitamins needed to obtain the same high blood levels as the 20 per cent of people with the lowest risk of coronary heart disease and cancer, the following intakes are obtained:

- Vitamin C   150 to 250 mg/day
- Vitamin E   50 to 100 mg/day
- Mixed carotenoids   15 mg/day
- Selenium   100 mcg/day

Other dietary antioxidants such as those found in blue-red berries (e.g. blueberries, grapes) and tea (especially green and white teas) are also thought to be important.

Smokers and people with diabetes need twice as many anti-oxidant vitamins as other people as they generate many more free radicals.

It is advisable to ensure a high dietary intake of vitamins C, E and betacarotene during pregnancy. As well as protecting our own health, the future health of the next generation is known to be linked with maternal dietary factors at the time of conception.

Recent studies suggest the development of coronary heart disease, stroke and diabetes in later years is linked to growth failure in the first few weeks of life. This in turn is linked to a deficient maternal diet. It may be that high blood levels of antioxidant vitamins protect the developing foetus from free radical attack enough to affect health in later life. This is not yet proved – but sensible supplementation can only do good.

7

Healthy eating for vegetarians and vegans

Vegetarians are usually very food aware and know exactly what constitutes a healthy, balanced diet. But a poor vegetarian diet can be just as bad as a poor omnivore diet if you don't know what you are doing.

It is the new vegetarian, who simply removes meat and/or dairy produce from their diet, without replacing it with other protein sources (often in a bid to eat more healthy), who is most at risk of nutritional imbalance. So long as alternative sources of protein (pulses, legumes, nuts, seeds, grains and cereals in place of meat) are obtained, the most likely deficiencies are of vitamin B12 and iron. Intakes of other nutrients (e.g. calcium and zinc) will depend on the type of vegetarian philosophy followed.

Vitamin D is found naturally in animal foods but is also synthesised in the skin when exposed to sunlight. Vegetarians who stay indoors a lot or who cover their skin in sunlight need to ensure an adequate intake of vitamin D and there is probably a case for taking dietary supplements.

There are several types of diet in which meats are excluded:

1. Those who don't eat certain meats (e.g. veal, pork) from certain animals. The remaining diet includes other meats and fish. No additional risk of a nutrient deficiency is incurred.

2. Those who don't eat meat, but do eat fish and dairy produce. This is a healthy eating option and there is little additional risk

of nutritional deficiency above that of the general population during pregnancy.

3. Those who don't eat meat or fish but do eat milk and eggs. This is called ovo-lacto-vegetarianism. This is the most common vegetarian lifestyle. The most frequently seen nutritional deficiency is lack of iron. Ovo-lacto-vegetarians miss out on the best sources of the most easily absorbed form of iron, haem iron (i.e. meat, fish), but this is partly compensated for by their higher intake of vitamin C. This improves absorption of non-haem iron from other sources. For example, when eating eggs, have a glass of freshly squeezed orange juice too. Women who are contemplating pregnancy are advised to ensure an adequate iron intake – through dietary changes or through supplementation. Some types of plant fibre, especially phytate, found in bran, decrease the absorption of minerals such as iron, zinc and calcium (see vegans, below). Lacto-ovo-vegetarians must also ensure their protein intake is adequate by eating plenty of pulses, legumes, nuts, seeds, grains and cereals. A personal nutritional analysis by a trained professional is recommended early on during their pre-conceptual care period.

4. Those who don't eat any meat or dairy products derived from animals. People following this regime are known as vegans. Vitamin B12 deficiency is almost universal without regular supplementation. As deficiency of vitamin B12 is associated with foetal abnormality (see page 66), supplementation is essential. Preparations of vitamin B12 that are made by bacterial fermentation – and are therefore ethically acceptable to vegetarians – are readily available.

   Other nutrients whose intakes are likely to be low include iron, calcium and zinc, as some types of fibre, especially phytate, decrease the absorption of these minerals.

   Those eating mainly vegetarian foods tend to obtain less than 66 per cent (and in some cases less than 50 per cent) of the recommended zinc intake. Vegans, with their traditional preference for wholemeal bread, could try calcium-enriched soya milk and include some white bread in their diet to counter the effects of their exceptionally high fibre intake. Either supplements or dietary changes to improve the intake of these nutrients are recommended.

Protein intake must be watched carefully – plenty of pulses, legumes, nuts, seeds, grains and cereals are essential.

All vegans should seek a personal nutritional analysis from a trained professional early on during their pre-conceptual care period. Multi-nutrient supplements should ideally be taken (see page 62).

5. Those who eat nothing but fruit. People following this regime are called fruitarians. This type of eating is not compatible with a healthy life if followed for any length of time. It is deficient in protein, complex carbohydrate, essential fatty acids, sodium, iron and vitamin B12 as well as many other vitamins and minerals. Fruitarianism cannot be recommended as a dietary philosophy during the pre-conceptual care period or pregnancy.

Recommendations for a healthy vegetarian diet

- Wholegrain cereals rather than refined cereals.
- Three to four servings of cereal and grains per day (e.g. bread, rice, pasta, buckwheat, polenta). These provide calories, protein, fibre, B vitamins, calcium and iron.
- At least 400 g vegetables/fruit per day in total (five portions), of which at least one is a citrus fruit for vitamin C.
- Dried fruits for fibre and iron.
- A large salad or portion of dark green, leafy vegetables (e.g. spinach, watercress, broccoli, greens) per day for folate, calcium and iron.
- Two large portions of carrots or sweet potato (yams) per week for protein, energy, fibre, calcium, iron, zinc and vitamin E. Aim for at least 30 g of pulses, seeds or nuts per day.
- Protein requirements increase to 50 g to 60 g per day during pregnancy. Nuts, seeds, pulses and cereals all contain protein

but none contains all the essential amino acids together – e.g. the essential amino acid missing from haricot beans is found in bread. Hence, combining cereals with pulses or seeds and nuts provides a balanced amino acid intake.

- Textured vegetable protein (TVP) made from soya beans is an excellent source of protein, calcium, iron, zinc, thiamine, riboflavin and niacin.
- Mycoprotein, derived from the fungus fusarium graminosum, is a good source of protein but is low in iron and calcium. Commercially available products tend to contain egg white, so are not suitable for vegans.
- One pint of semi-skimmed milk (or fortified soya milk) per day for protein, calcium and minerals.
- A serving (at least 60 g) of cheese per day for protein, calcium and minerals.
- A total of three or four eggs per week.
- Aim to eat no more than 30 per cent of total calories as fat. Less than 10 per cent of calories should be saturated fat (i.e. avoid excessive pastries, quiches, peanuts, crisps, coconut).
- Aim to eat no less than 20 per cent of calories as fat – ideally including plenty of olive oil and nut oils. Consider taking evening primrose oil if your intake of nuts and seeds is low.
- Some vegetable oils, margarine or butter for vitamins D and E.
- Adequate vitamin B12 levels, e.g. fortified soya milk, fortified breakfast cereals, fortified yeast extracts, Protoveg or supplements.

8

Body weight and pre-conceptual care

A woman's body weight and, more importantly, where her excess fat is preferentially stored is linked to her chance of a successful conception, a healthy pregnancy and a healthy, normal-weight baby.

Fat distribution

One study has shown that apple-shaped women are more likely to have difficulty in becoming pregnant than those who are pear-shaped. Waist and hip measurements were taken for 542 women attending a fertility clinic in Holland. All were of normal fertility but were attending for artificial insemination due to the reduced fertility of their partners.

The waist to hip ratio for each woman was calculated, with a ratio greater than 0.85 counting as high (apple-shaped) and a ratio less than 0.7 counting as low (more pear-shaped). Here are two examples:

$$\text{Waist:} \quad \frac{65 \text{ cm}}{95 \text{ cm}} = \text{ratio } 0.68$$
$$\text{Hip:}$$

$$\text{Waist:} \quad \frac{87 \text{ cm}}{100 \text{ cm}} = 0.87$$
$$\text{Hip:}$$

The women then underwent intracervical insemination procedures during subsequent menstrual cycles. The researchers compared the number of cycles to first conception with the women's waist to hip ratios and found that apple-shaped women were most likely to have difficulty conceiving.

An increase of just 0.1 in the waist to hip ratio led to a 30 per cent decrease in the probability of conception, regardless of the patient's age, overall weight, menstrual cycle characteristics or smoking habits.

The cumulative pregnancy rate for women with a waist to hip ratio less than 0.8 (pear-shaped) was 63 per cent compared with 32 per cent for women with a ratio greater than 0.8 (apple-shaped).

Although the women were partners of infertile men, because artificial insemination was used, the researchers argued that the results apply to the general population.

Working out if you are an apple or a pear

Using a non-stretch paper tape measure, work out both your waist and hip measurements accurately at rest – don't hold your tummy in! You can use either centimetres or inches so long as the same measurement is taken for both readings. Now divide your waist measurement by your hip measurement to get the ratio.

$$\frac{\text{Waist}}{\text{Hip}} = \text{Ratio}$$

If the ratio is greater than 0.85 for women (0.95 for men), you are an apple or android shape. If your ratio is less, you are a pear or gynoid shape.

Your waist to hip ratio is important to your general health too. Apple-shaped people are at greater risk of coronary heart disease, stroke, high blood pressure, atherosclerosis (furring up of the arteries), high blood cholesterol and diabetes than those with a more peripheral, pear-shaped distribution of fat. The reason for this is not fully understood, but may be related to altered metabolism of a special type of fat (brown fat) found in certain parts of the body.

Obesity and pre-conceptual care

The number of overweight women is increasing, making obesity one of the most common high-risk conditions in obstetrics. In the US, for example, as many as 38 per cent of pregnant women in some surveys were obese.

Any excess fat you carry during the pre-conceptual care period is likely to increase significantly during pregnancy itself due to the changing hormone environment, especially high levels of progesterone.

Pregnancy is a liberating experience for many overweight women. After a lifetime of embarrassment about their appearance, they at last have an excuse for overeating – and can even feel proud of their girth. Being overweight is a socially acceptable condition if a woman is pregnant and can lead to greatly improved self-esteem.

In one study of 37 overweight women, all of whom weighed at least 90 kg (14 stone) when 30 weeks pregnant, 41 per cent felt more self-confident about their weight than they had before they were pregnant. But six weeks after giving birth, they all felt negative with low self-esteem – and little motivation to tackle their burgeoning weight.

It is important not to fall into this trap. Overweight women tend to put on much more weight during pregnancy than normal-weight women. All their bad eating habits strike with a vengeance because, for once, it is acceptable to overeat.

Average weight gain during pregnancy is 10 to 12.5 kg (22 to 28 lb). Any more than this is excessive and potentially hazardous, especially in women who are obese to start with. It increases the likelihood of:

- A large baby (foetal macrosomia).
- A difficult labour.
- Developing high blood pressure.
- Gestational diabetes.
- Post-maturity (overdue by more than 2 weeks) of the foetus.
- Having an induced labour.

Overweight (BMI 25–30 or weight 120–150 per cent of ideal body weight) increases the risk of developing gestational diabetes by 1.8 to 6.5 times. In women classed as obese (BMI >30 or weight >150 per cent of ideal body weight), the incidence of gestational diabetes is 1.4- to 20-fold higher than for those in the healthy weight range for their height.

High blood pressure and pre-eclampsia are also more common, with those who are obese being 2.2 to 21.4 times more likely to have high blood pressure, and 1.22 to 9.7 times more likely to develop pre-eclampsia.

Obesity during pregnancy also increases the chance of urinary tract infections and of developing abnormal blood clotting problems. The only benefit appears to be that anaemia is less common in severely obese pregnant women compared with those of healthy weight.

Being overweight also increases the chance of needing a Caesarean section by a factor of 1.5 to 3 times. The usual reasons are a large baby which is difficult to deliver vaginally, foetal distress and failure of labour to progress. A recent study of 167,750 pregnant women also found that obesity increased the frequency of very premature delivery (<32 weeks) but only during a first pregnancy. For those who had previously had a baby, obesity did not seem to be a significant risk factor for premature delivery.

For the offspring of overweight women, there appears to be an increased risk of neural tube defect and other congenital abnormalities. Data based on 56,857 children in the US found that major congenital malformations were 35 per cent more common in the offspring of mothers who were overweight and 37.5 per cent more likely in those classed as obese. Neural tube defects were 1.8 to 3 times more common in the offspring of overweight women, even when maternal age, smoking and folic acid intake were accounted for. Recent studies have also shown that overweight and obese women were 3.3 times more likely than healthy-weight women to have an infant with an umbilical abnormality, twice as likely to have a child with a heart defect and twice as likely to have a child with multiple developmental abnormalities.

Other problems that are more likely in the offspring include large size (making delivery difficult), breathing problems and low Apgar score after delivery, and undescended testicles in male infants (2.4 times more common in those born to obese mums).

Sadly, the babies of overweight women are up to 2.5 times more likely to die in the two weeks after birth, and those of obese women are 3.4 times more likely to succumb.

Other studies have shown that losing weight can restore normal menstrual cycle regularity and increase your chances of conception.

It is advisable to lose any excess weight as part of your pre-conceptual programme before you try to conceive. Apart from increasing your chances of conception, a normal weight increases the chance of a healthy pregnancy, problem-free labour and a healthy, normal-weight baby. Watch your weight during pregnancy too, and don't eat for two!

How to work out if you need to lose weight

The most modern way of estimating excess body fat is the body mass index (BMI). There is a more or less constant relationship between weight and the square of a person's height:

$$BMI = \frac{Weight\ (kg)}{Height\ (m) \times Height\ (m)}$$

BMI is used to grade body fat content as follows:

Body mass index (kg/m^2)	Weight band	Grade
<18.7	Underweight	–
18.7–25	Healthy	0
25–30	Overweight	I
30–40	Obese	II
>40	Morbidly obese	III

NB This does not apply if you are already pregnant.

BODY MASS INDEX READY RECKONER

HEIGHT – feet and inches (across)   **WEIGHT –** (down the side; scale shown in stones 19–13 with intermediate pound marks 12, 10, 8, 6, 4, 2, 0)

WEIGHT	4'6"	4'8"	4'10"	5'0"	5'2"	5'4"	5'6"	5'8"	5'10"	6'0"	6'2"	6'4"	6'6"
125	66	62	58	54	50	47	44	42	40	37	35	34	32
124	66	61	57	53	50	47	44	42	39	37	35	33	32
123	65	61	57	53	50	47	44	41	39	37	35	33	31
122	65	60	56	53	49	46	43	41	39	37	35	33	31
121	64	60	56	52	49	46	43	41	38	36	34	33	31
120	64	59	55	52	48	45	43	40	38	36	34	32	31
119	63	59	55	51	48	45	42	40	38	36	34	32	30
118	63	58	54	51	48	45	42	40	37	35	33	32	30
117	62	58	54	50	47	44	42	39	37	35	33	31	30
116	62	57	53	50	47	44	41	39	37	35	33	31	30
115	61	57	53	50	46	44	41	39	36	34	33	31	29
114	61	56	53	49	46	43	41	38	36	34	32	31	29
113	60	56	52	49	46	43	40	38	36	34	32	30	29
112	60	55	52	48	45	42	40	38	35	34	32	30	29
111	59	55	51	48	45	42	40	37	35	33	31	30	28
110	58	54	51	47	44	42	39	37	35	33	31	30	28
109	58	54	50	47	44	41	39	37	34	33	31	29	28
108	57	53	50	47	44	41	38	36	34	32	31	29	28
107	57	53	49	46	43	41	38	36	34	32	30	29	27
106	56	52	49	46	43	40	38	36	34	32	30	28	27
105	56	52	48	45	42	40	37	35	33	31	30	28	27
104	55	51	48	45	42	39	37	35	33	31	29	28	27
103	55	51	47	44	42	39	37	35	33	31	29	28	26
102	54	50	47	44	41	39	36	34	32	31	29	27	26
101	54	50	47	44	41	38	36	34	32	30	29	27	26
100	53	49	46	43	40	38	36	34	32	30	28	27	26
99	53	49	46	43	40	38	35	33	31	30	28	27	25
98	52	48	45	42	40	37	35	33	31	29	28	26	25
97	52	48	45	42	39	37	35	33	31	29	28	26	25
96	51	47	44	41	39	36	34	32	30	29	27	26	25
95	51	47	44	41	38	36	34	32	30	28	27	26	24
94	50	46	43	40	38	36	33	32	30	28	27	25	24
93	49	46	43	40	38	35	33	31	29	28	26	25	24
92	49	45	42	40	37	35	33	31	29	28	26	25	23
91	48	45	42	39	37	34	32	31	29	27	26	24	23
90	48	44	41	39	36	34	32	30	29	27	26	24	23
89	47	44	41	38	36	34	32	30	28	27	25	24	23
88	47	43	41	38	36	33	31	30	28	26	25	24	22
87	46	43	40	37	35	33	31	29	28	26	25	23	22
86	46	43	40	37	35	33	31	29	27	26	24	23	22

WEIGHT –

stones

HEIGHT – metres

WEIGHT

HEIGHT

kilograms

Used with the permission of Servier Laboratories (UK) Limited

For non-pregnant women, a BMI in the range of 20–25 kg/m^2 is the healthiest. Women with a BMI above 30 kg/m^2 are in the obese range and more likely to have difficulty conceiving or problems during pregnancy – as are women with a BMI under 20 kg/m^2. Being underweight is just as unhealthy as being overweight.

Use the mass index chart on pages 114 and 115 to compute your BMI by plotting your height in metres against your weight in kilograms. The squaring is automatically calculated for you.

Using the body mass index, it's possible to work backwards and calculate a range of desirable, healthy weights to aim for during the pre-conceptual care period.

Optimum body weight for non-pregnant women (based on BMI of 18.7–25)

Height		Optimum body weight range	
Metres	*Feet*	*Kg*	*Stones*
1.47	4' 10"	40–54	6st 4–8st 7
1.50	4' 11"	42–56	6st 8–8st 11
1.52	5 ft	43–58	6st 11–9st 2
1.55	5' 1"	45–60	7st 1–9st 7
1.57	5' 2"	46–62	7st 3–9st 11
1.60	5' 3"	48–64	7st 8–10st 1
1.63	5' 4"	50–66	7st 12–10st 6
1.65	5' 5"	51–68	8st–10st 10
1.68	5' 6"	53–70	8st 5–11st
1.70	5' 7"	54–72	8st 7–11st 4
1.73	5' 8"	56–75	8st 11–11st 10
1.75	5' 9"	57–76	8st 13–12 st
1.78	5' 10"	59–79	9st 4–12st 6
1.80	5' 11"	61–81	9st 8–12st 9
1.83	6 ft	63–83	9st 13–13st 1

125 – [67]

Losing weight safely in the pre-conceptual care period

It is important to lose weight sensibly and slowly during the pre-conceptual care period. The common practice of going on a crash diet is particularly dangerous within a few weeks or months of conceiving.

Apart from an increased risk of miscarriage classic diets involve cutting down on high-fat dairy products such as butter, whole milk, cream and cheese. These are an important source of calcium. Calcium requirements are increased during pregnancy and it is important that you don't cut out these products altogether. A varied diet, providing all the vitamins, minerals, fibre, carbo-hydrate, protein and essential fats you need but without the excess calories is important. Drink a pint of semi-skimmed milk per day as part of your calorie allowance.

It is best not to be obsessed with slimming during this important period of your life. If you are very overweight (BMI greater than 30 kg/m^2) seek professional advice from your doctor or a dietician. Otherwise, follow a modified Mediterranean-style healthy eating plan (see page 45) and increase the amount of exercise you take.

Aim for a daily energy intake of 1,200 to 1,500 kcals and you will find you naturally lose weight slowly at a rate of around 0.5 to 1 kg (1 to 2 lb) per week. Losing weight any faster than this will put the health of your future baby at risk. Under-nourishment during the first few weeks of life (due to poor maternal diet) is increasingly linked with the development of serious disease in later life (see page 43). You will need to ensure an adequate intake of vitamins and minerals – a multi-nutrient is an excellent idea if you are curbing your dietary intake.

Healthy slimming tips

- Cut down on the amount of butter you eat. Try a reduced-fat spread made with olive oil.
- Switch to low-fat brands of salad dressing, cheese, milk, yoghurt, etc.

- Use lemon juice or yoghurt instead of oily salad dressing or salad cream.
- Drink a pint of semi-skimmed milk per day – it contains as much calcium and protein as full-fat milk.
- Use low-fat yoghurt or fromage frais instead of cream or custard.
- Eat less red meat – three times per week or less is better than the more usual once or twice per day.
- Eat more lean white meat (e.g. chicken).
- Cut skin and visible fat from meat and discard it.
- Eat more fish – at least twice a week.
- Fill up on bread, pasta, rice and plain potatoes – obtain at least half your daily energy from these.
- Eat five portions of fruit or vegetables per day.
- Have regular vegetarian days.
- Eat 30 g nuts or seeds per day when cutting down on red meat.
- Cut out cakes, chips, biscuits, crisps and chocolate.
- Grill, steam, poach or casserole food rather than frying or roasting.
- Eat baked potatoes rather than roasted or chipped.
- Drink plenty of mineral water or fruit/herbal teas instead of sweetened or fizzy drinks.
- Don't add salt to food – use fresh herbs for flavour.
- Only eat when you are hungry.
- Eat little and often – e.g. six small meals spread throughout the day rather than three large meals at set times.
- Avoid alcohol.
- Exercise briskly (e.g. walking, cycling, swimming) for at least 20 minutes, three times per week.

Underweight women

If your BMI is less than 18.7 kg/m^2 you are definitely underweight and more likely to have difficulty conceiving than normal-weight women, with fewer resources for you and your baby to draw on during pregnancy itself. In one study of 575 non-smoking women in their first pregnancy, growth of the developing baby increased as the mother's BMI increased, up to a BMI of 22–23 kg/m^2. Babies born to the women who were severely underweight before pregnancy (less than BMI 18.5 kg/m^2) were 80 per cent more likely to have growth problems within the womb. Being moderately underweight (BMI between 18.5 and 19.8 kg/m^2) was not significantly associated with adverse outcomes, however. Women who are severely underweight are usually advised to try to put on weight before becoming pregnant where possible.

Eating disorders

Eating disorders are emotional conditions in which food intake becomes extreme: either too much is eaten (bulimia nervosa) or too little (anorexia nervosa).

Ninety per cent of cases affect females and the majority start during the teens or early twenties. Approximately one in 150 girls aged 15 to 18 suffers from anorexia and 1 per cent to 2 per cent of women between 18 and 25 years of age suffer bulimia.

Both conditions, though especially bulimia, are characterised by self-induced vomiting and abuse of laxatives, diuretics or purgatives. These practices are harmful during pregnancy and can also result in subfertility.

If you have suffered from an eating disorder in the past, or are suffering now, it is vital that you seek help early on during your pre-conceptual care programme. There is evidence that offspring born to mothers with a history of eating disorders subsequently develop disturbed eating patterns themselves. This is probably a learned, behavioural event but there is evidence from twin studies of an hereditary component.

Anorexia

Anorexia nervosa is characterised by a morbid fear of fatness, a distorted body image and a relentless pursuit of thinness. It mainly affects young women of reproductive age (13 to 30) of whom a third have previously been overweight. In effect, dieting has become obsessive.

Undereating, with some women only consuming 200 kcals per

day or less, leads to rapid and excessive weight loss. Dehydration, salt and acid imbalances and gross nutritional deficiencies of protein, carbohydrate, fibre, essential fatty acids, vitamins (especially B12 and folate) and minerals also occur. These increase the risk of foetal malnutrition and developmental abnormalities such as neural tube defect and hare lip in the unlikely event that pregnancy occurs.

As soon as body weight plummets below a certain point, menstruation stops and infertility starts. The body is physically incapable of maintaining a pregnancy. The ovaries and uterus thin right down. One study of 26 anorexics showed they had an average uterine volume of 5.5 cubic centimetres, compared with an expected volume of 15 cc.

Anorexics usually have low levels of all minerals, but especially calcium, copper, magnesium, iron, selenium and zinc. Because of a lack of dietary calcium, anorexics can lose bone mass at a rate of 15 per cent in a single year. Bone density only increases at a rate of 1 per cent to 2 per cent per year once relatively normal eating patterns resume. This means there is an increased risk of future pregnancy-associated osteoporosis.

Anorexics are grossly zinc deficient – whether this is a cause or effect observation is still hotly in dispute. Some researchers suggest that zinc supplementation can improve the food intake of 85 per cent of anorexics as it restores taste sensation.

For a healthy, safe pregnancy, normal eating patterns, weight, hydration and electrolyte imbalances need to be restored. Vitamin and mineral supplements are essential. Recovery from anorexia nervosa requires a slow process of psychological and physical rehabilitation to correct the underlying distorted self-image and self-esteem.

Bulimia

Bulimics have many of the psychological features of anorexia but alternate periods of starvation with massive binges. They are capable of eating as many as 42,000 kcals in 24 hours. These are subsequently disgorged upwards, usually through self-induced vomiting.

A third of bulimics have a history of anorexia nervosa and a few have co-existent anorexia. These patients have a worse prognosis than those suffering from bulimia alone.

Bulimia is recognised as a serious, under-diagnosed, long-term and potentially fatal illness. It can be successfully treated using cognitive, behavioural, educational and insight-orientated psycho-therapy approaches.

If bulimia is diagnosed during pregnancy, it is treated early, vigorously and preferably without the use of drugs. An increasing number of women are known to develop bulimia in the first three months of pregnancy – often in an attempt not to put on weight. It is easy to confuse this with morning sickness.

The metabolic effects (salt and acid imbalances) of induced vomiting increase the risk of miscarriage, pre-term delivery and obstetric complications. In addition, nutritional deficiencies result in foetal abnormalities such as cleft palate and cleft (hare) lip.

It is vitally important that affected women seek help – ideally during the pre-conceptual care period, but help at any stage during pregnancy is better than suffering alone. Studies suggest that some untreated bulimics improve during pregnancy but usually relapse after delivery.

Bulimics are also putting themselves at risk of long-term infertility from a condition called polycystic ovary syndrome, even if their weight is normal. Ultrasound studies of 34 bulimics showed that only four (12 per cent) had normal ovaries while 30 (88 per cent) women had polycystic or multi-follicular ovaries. It is thought that these ovarian changes are due to insulin resistance induced by fluctuating blood sugar levels between starving and bingeing. It is not yet known whether the ovaries return to normal once eating behaviour is corrected.

Polycystic ovaries are associated with scanty or absent periods, infertility and excessive body hair. The condition is usually caused by an imbalance between two hormones secreted by the pituitary gland – luteinising hormone (LH) and follicle stimulating hormone (FSH). This results in lack of ovulation, the formation of ovarian cysts and increased production of the male hormone testosterone.

9

Exercise

The number of women who remain physically active during pregnancy is increasing, partly because women feel that exercise has a positive influence on their pregnancy experience, and partly because of the increased availability of pre-natal exercise classes (e.g. aerobics, swimming). Most studies agree that the benefits of exercise during pregnancy outweigh the risks.

An interesting study published in 2003 studied fourteen women before, during and for six months after a planned pregnancy to see how their bodies responded to the increased oxygen demands of exercise during pregnancy. The women took part in a bicycle exercise test in which they reached a target heart rate of 85 per cent of their predicted maximum (220 beats/min minus age in years). The amount of oxygen their blood could carry (oxygen saturation) was found to have increased significantly as early as 8 weeks' gestation, and continued to increase until 29 weeks of gestation when it started to fall, so that by 36 weeks' gestation it was just above the pre-pregnancy value. This suggests that, during pregnancy, women can maintain and even increase the oxygen supply to their tissues during short-term exercise during the first 29 weeks. Interestingly, their core body temperature reduced during exercise as their pregnancy progressed, from a pre-conception level of 37.8 degrees C to post-partum levels of 36.9 degrees C. This suggests that the body has a way of reducing the temperature response to exercise during pregnancy as excess heat is known to be harmful to a developing baby.

It is important to get into the peak of fitness during your pre-conceptual care programme. Inactivity before and during pregnancy can encourage a sluggish metabolism, weight gain, high blood pressure, high blood cholesterol levels and poor handling of body glucose.

In addition, lack of exercise causes lethargy, makes you feel tired all the time and can encourage depression. Worst of all, it can lower your sex drive, which is not ideal – especially during the pre-conceptual care programme! Unexercised muscles are flabby, joints seize up and ligaments stiffen – all of which make late pregnancy uncomfortable and labour more prolonged.

In contrast, regular physical exercise has positive effects on health for both men and women, especially during the pre-conceptual care period.

The benefits of a pre-conceptual exercise programme

Regular exercise curbs your appetite, boosts your metabolic rate and imparts a wonderful feeling of energy. In addition, exercise:

- Improves your strength, stamina and suppleness.
- Reduces high blood cholesterol levels.
- Reduces high blood pressure.
- Speeds up the metabolism and burns fat.
- Tones up muscles, including abdominal ones, and firms your silhouette.
- Improves the efficiency of your heart.
- Strengthens your bones and decreases the risk of osteoporosis.
- Generates feelings of euphoria.
- Improves your self-esteem.

It is important not to overdo exercise, however. Excessive training can significantly lower fertility in men (see page 221).

How to walk yourself fit

Brisk walking is an excellent, low-impact exercise for building up fitness both before and during pregnancy, especially if you've been relatively inactive over the last year. Brisk walking burns up over 350 calories per hour – more if you swing your arms and put extra effort into it – and can help a sensible weight-loss programme.

A walking for fitness programme involves brisk, regular walks, not infrequent leisurely strolls. Make sure you wear recommended shoes with cushioned soles and some ankle support. Warm up first with a few simple stretch exercises. Begin slowly and lengthen your strides as you go.

You should soon feel warm and start to generate a light sweat. Don't let yourself feel out of breath to the extent that you can't walk and talk at the same time. After your brisk walk, stroll gently for a few minutes to cool down, then do some simple stretch exercises to maintain muscle suppleness.

A suggested walking for fitness regime is given below. Obviously you don't need to stick to the days of the week suggested but try to spread your activity evenly throughout the week.

Suggested pre-conceptual walking regime

Week	Monday	Wednesday	Friday	Sunday
1	10 mins	10 mins	15 mins	
2	10 mins	10 mins	15 mins	
3	10 mins	15 mins	15 mins	
4	15 mins	15 mins	15 mins	15 mins
5	15 mins	15 mins	20 mins	20 mins
6	20 mins	20 mins	25 mins	25 mins
7	25 mins	25 mins	25 mins	25 mins
8	30 mins	30 mins	30 mins	30 mins
9	30 mins	35 mins	30 mins	35 mins
10	40 mins	35 mins	40 mins	35 mins
11	40 mins	40 mins	40 mins	40 mins
12	45 mins	40 mins	45 mins	40 mins

To maintain your new fitness level, continue walking briskly three or four times per week. Try to obtain at least 20–30 minutes' exercise three times per week.

Exercise during pregnancy itself

It is safe to continue a regular fitness programme during pregnancy. The fitter you are and the stronger your abdominal muscles, the easier you'll find the demands of late pregnancy and labour.

Fears about exercise causing miscarriage are often voiced soon after conception is confirmed, but many doctors now believe the traditional advice for mothers to take excessive rest is unnecessary. There is no firm evidence to suggest that moderate exercise results in foetal harm or pre-term birth, but do not take up a new sport during pregnancy.

Non-weight-bearing exercises such as swimming or cycling are particularly good as they improve strength, stamina and suppleness without stressing the joints.

From the fourth month of pregnancy onwards, avoid high-impact sports such as jogging, sprinting or advanced aerobics and activities such as skiing or horse-riding where falling is a possibility.

As pregnancy progresses, you will start to tire more easily. Your ligaments, including those in your back and pelvis, will start to slacken due to the effects of progesterone and a hormone known as relaxin. As a result, joint aches and pains can become problematic and you are more susceptible to joint strains or even tears.

Avoid exercising flat on your back – as is common in aerobics and keep-fit classes – from the fifth month onwards. This can affect your circulation and cause dizziness. You should also avoid strong stomach muscle exercises from five months onwards as these are already stretched to accommodate the foetus. Further stretching may do more harm than good. The time to build up your stomach muscles is during the pre-conceptual care programme and early pregnancy.

The best advice is to start tapering off your exercise levels from the sixth month of pregnancy onwards. In any case, the increasing bulk of your breasts and abdomen will naturally curtail your activities.

The simple rule to follow is: if you feel uncomfortable or tired, STOP. Never let yourself get out of breath.

10

General health screening during pre-conceptual care

Early on in your pre-conceptual care programme, it is important to attend a well woman or designated pre-conceptual clinic for a health check-up. A full, pre-conceptual care screening will ensure that:

- You are protected against rubella (German measles).
- You do not have high blood pressure.
- You do not have albumin (protein) or glucose (sugar) in your urine.
- You have a normal, healthy cervical smear.
- You do not have a vaginal infection.
- You are not excessively over- or underweight.
- You are following a healthy lifestyle and diet including any necessary vitamin or mineral supplements as recommended by your doctor.

Screening for rubella

Rubella (German measles) is a relatively innocuous viral illness *unless* it is contracted during the early months of pregnancy. It can then cause devastating birth defects known as Rubella Syndrome.

Rubella is contracted from person to person by airborne droplets containing infectious viral particles. Symptoms develop after an incubation period of two to three weeks.

In children and adults, rubella causes a mild rash on the face which spreads to the trunk and limbs. This usually disappears within a few days. There is sometimes a slight fever and enlargement of lymph nodes (glands) at the back of the neck. Sometimes the illness passes unnoticed, although adults usually fair worse, with headache, a higher fever and sometimes inflammation of the joints.

However, rubella is dangerous to the unborn child if the mother contracts it during the first four months of pregnancy. If it is contracted during the first few weeks of pregnancy, there is a greater than 50 per cent chance that the foetus will be affected. During the third month of pregnancy, the risk is 17 per cent, but from the fourth month onwards the risk is negligible. Generally, the earlier rubella is contracted in pregnancy, the more seriously the foetus is affected. Congenital Rubella Syndrome in the foetus is associated with:

- Miscarriage.
- Deafness.
- Heart defects.
- Mental retardation.
- Cataracts, eye defects and blindness.
- Skin bruising (purpura).
- Cerebral palsy.
- Bone deformities.
- Facial abnormalities.
- Stillbirth.
- A 20 per cent risk of dying during early infancy.
- Continued shedding of rubella virus in urine, faeces and saliva for up to a year after birth.

As a result of rubella immunisation programmes, the disease is now less common.

Rubella Syndrome is entirely preventable. During the pre-conceptual care period, all women should have a blood test to assess their level of anti-rubella antibodies. This should be done even if you know you have previously had the disease or received inoculation. It is possible for antibody levels to fall so that you are no longer protected.

Any woman whose antibody levels are inadequate should be vaccinated *before* becoming pregnant. The vaccine is contra-indicated during pregnancy itself as it contains live, inactivated virus. This may occasionally activate to give rise to mild symptoms of the disease and affect the foetus itself (see page 152). Contra-ceptive measures should be taken during vaccination and for twelve weeks afterwards. After inoculation, your antibody levels should be checked by a subsequent blood test to ensure protection.

It is wise for all women who are pregnant, or planning to be, to avoid contact with any person who is ill or has a rash to minimise the risks of infection. If a non-immune woman who is or might be pregnant comes into contact with anyone thought to have rubella, she should immediately seek medical advice. Passive immunisation with antibodies (immunoglobulins) may help prevent infection of the foetus.

Screening for high blood pressure

High blood pressure increases the risks during pregnancy of miscarriage, kidney problems, strokes, etc. Any woman who has high blood pressure during the pre-conceptual care period will need a thorough medical investigation to find the cause. Medication may be advised to control your blood pressure before you attempt to conceive. You will also require regular medical attention through-out the pregnancy itself.

Screening for sugar diabetes

Women who suffer from diabetes have a metabolic disorder characterised by a relative lack of insulin – a hormone needed to help body cells take up glucose and use it for energy.

It is important to be screened for diabetes before becoming pregnant. This is easily done at your general practice surgery by dipping a reagent strip into a sample of your urine. If any sugar is present, you will need a full medical investigation and treatment to stabilise your blood sugar control before attempting to conceive.

Mild forms of diabetes are treated by diet and in some cases oral medication which lowers blood sugar. Insulin will probably be required at some stage during pregnancy. More severe forms of the disease require regular insulin injections throughout life, with particular care taken during pregnancy itself.

Approximately 1 per cent to 2 per cent of pregnant women have diabetes. Many hospitals offer pre-conceptual care clinics especially for diabetic women. Throughout your pregnancy, you will usually be cared for by both an obstetrician and a physician specialising in diabetes. Nearly all women with established diabetes are able to have a successful pregnancy, but pre-conceptual care, a planned pregnancy, careful monitoring and tight control of blood sugar levels throughout are essential. Otherwise, complications are possible, such as:

- Cystitis and thrush.
- Kidney problems.
- Placental insufficiency.
- Excess amniotic fluid.
- Pre-eclampsia (a serious disease of pregnancy, in which high blood pressure, fluid accumulation and protein in the urine develop).
- Eclampsia (an advanced form of pre-eclampsia in which fitting occurs).
- A build-up of acid and toxins in the body (ketoacidosis).
- A large baby.
- A difficult labour.
- Instrumental delivery (forceps, Caesarean).
- Stillbirth.
- Babies with congenital abnormalities.

This is quite a frightening list, but most problems are successfully avoided by paying strict attention to sugar control and attending for all necessary antenatal check-ups.

Around 5 per cent of non-diabetic women develop diabetes as a result of pregnancy. This is known as gestational diabetes. It tends to appear during the second half of pregnancy and usually resolves once the pregnancy is over.

Gestational diabetes is more common in women over the age of 25, those with a family history of diabetes, those who put on a lot of weight during pregnancy and those carrying a large baby. Your antenatal care will involve regular repeat testing of your urine to check for unexpected sugar.

Diabetics have a marked reduction in blood vitamin C levels compared with non-diabetic controls – despite no obvious difference in dietary intake. Some experts recommend that diabetics, especially if they smoke, should take vitamin C supplements – perhaps in dosages as high as 500 mg per day. In general, diabetics need twice as many antioxidant vitamins as non-diabetics to mop up the additional free radicals generated by their abnormal metabolic reactions (see page 101).

No special precautions other than a sensible control of blood sugar levels are required by a diabetic man planning to become a father. Interestingly, there is evidence that sperm from diabetic men are more fertile than usual. Their sperm seem to swim in straighter lines (see page 219).

The chance of a baby with one diabetic parent developing diabetes throughout life is around one in 100. If both parents are diabetic, the risk increases to one in 20.

Screening for protein in the urine

The presence of albumin protein in your urine (albuminuria) should be checked for during the pre-conceptual care period. Trace amounts of albumin are usually nothing to worry about, although further tests may be advised.

If moderate to large amounts of albumin are detected in your urine, this suggests kidney disease or a urinary tract infection. You will need full screening tests to assess the anatomy and functioning of your kidneys before getting the go-ahead to try for conception.

Vaginal and pelvic health

Cervical smears

Cervical screening is basically an early warning system. It is designed to detect early cell changes which, if left untreated, may develop into cancer at some stage in the future. Cervical smears every three to five years help to screen for early changes. If you are in any doubt as to whether you need a smear, or when your last one was performed, make it a priority to contact your doctor and find out.

If you are due a cervical smear, request one early on during your pre-conceptual care period and wait for the all-clear before attempting to conceive. Smears are best taken mid-menstrual cycle where possible.

Women below the age of 25 years who started sexual activity at an early age (before 18 years old), or who've had multiple sexual partners, should also seek a cervical smear during their pre-conceptual care period. If abnormalities are found, try not to panic. In most cases, these are mild to moderate changes which only need regular monitoring. They may well revert to normal without treatment. More severe changes will need examination under a special microscope (colposcope) and a small biopsy to see if further treatment is indicated. The cervix may then be treated with diathermy (electrical heat) or laser therapy to kill abnormal cells before you attempt conception.

Abnormalities cannot be properly investigated or treated during pregnancy. In addition, the hormonal changes that occur during pregnancy may affect cervical cells. It is much safer to have any necessary treatment carried out before you become pregnant than to have to wait until your baby is born. If you are told your smear shows inflammation or abnormalities, find out exactly what is wrong and what implications this has for your future planned pregnancy.

11

Female genital infections

Many vaginal or pelvic infections exist without obvious early symptoms. As pelvic infection increases your risk of subfertility, miscarriage, pre-term delivery and infection of your future child, some specialists recommend having a vaginal health check-up during the pre-conceptual care period. This involves a quick visual examination, the taking of swabs and examination of fresh vaginal discharge under a microscope.

A genito-urinary check-up is especially important if you notice:

- Any abnormality of your vaginal discharge, e.g. increased quantity, unusual smell or staining.
- Itching, soreness, tenderness or pain.
- Abnormal bleeding.
- Lumps or ulceration.
- Pain on urinating (dysuria, cystitis).
- Low abdominal pain.
- Discomfort during intercourse.
- Genital problems in your regular partner.
- And if you are at risk of having contracted a sexually transmitted disease.

Your vaginal health check is best carried out in a specialist genito-urinary medicine (GUM) clinic. These have the advantage over many GP surgeries in that they examine fresh discharge under a microscope and can pick up most bacterial imbalances or diseases there and then. Sending a vaginal swab to hospital for culture and microscopy often proves unhelpful. Few bugs survive well enough to be detected several days later and mild (yet important) infections or bacterial imbalances are frequently missed.

Microscopy of fresh vaginal discharge plus sophisticated tests in the laboratory will help to exclude or confirm vaginal infections – not all of which are necessarily sexually transmissible.

The common, important genito-urinary infections are discussed individually below.

Candida (thrush)

Thrush is a common vaginal pathogen (organism that causes disease) caused by a microscopic, yeast-like fungus, candida albicans.

Infection is sometimes without symptoms but more usually results in itching, soreness, pain on intercourse, dryness and a white, cottage-cheese-like discharge. The quantity of discharge does not necessarily equate with the severity of symptoms.

Thrush spores are present in the air and germinate in warm, moist places. Candida thrives when natural immunity falls during times of stress and illness, or when antibiotics destroy the normal vaginal bacteria that help keep yeast infections at bay.

Women taking the oral contraceptive Pill, who are pregnant, or in the second half of their menstrual cycle (post-ovulation) have high oestrogen levels which increase the glycogen (sugar) content of their vaginal cells. Together with the falling acidity of secretions that also occurs at these times, their chance of developing thrush increases. Some women seem to develop thrush regularly, possibly because of a reservoir of infection in their gut. Recurrent thrush may be associated with iron-deficiency anaemia, low blood ferritin (molecules carrying iron in the blood) levels and sugar diabetes, for which your GP will screen you.

Topical creams and pre-filled syringes of vaginal preparations are available from pharmacies or on prescription. These topical treatments are safe during the pre-conceptual care period and during pregnancy.

For women who suffer regular infection, oral medication to eradicate candida from the bowel may be prescribed. Oral treatments cannot be used during pregnancy. Women who are prescribed them during their pre-conceptual care programme must ensure they use adequate contraception during treatment and for at least one month following.

Self-help remedies for vaginal thrush include:

- Taking probiotic supplements (containing friendly bacteria such as Lactobacilli).
- Avoiding bath washes, vaginal deodorants or douches. All destroy the protective acid mantle of the vagina. Those containing lactic acid are acceptable.
- Wearing loose clothing with cotton gussets. Tights, nylon panties and close-fitting trousers all increase warmth and humidity in the groin, increasing the risk of thrush infection.
- Hot-ironing panty gussets. Modern low-temperature washing machine cycles don't always kill candida spores and re-infection can occur from your own underwear.
- Your partner should ideally be treated with an anti-thrush cream too, to reduce the risk of passing infection back to you when you next make love.

Anaerobic vaginosis

Most bacteria living in your vagina need oxygen to survive and are therefore classified as aerobic. A minority of vaginal bacteria are anaerobic, preferring low levels of oxygen saturation.

Bacterial imbalances frequently occur when anaerobes over-grow and oust the protective, aerobic bacteria. This causes an increased, smelly discharge often accompanied by soreness (anaerobic bacterial vaginosis).

Recent studies suggest that bacterial vaginosis accounts for up to 50 per cent of all vaginal infections in non-pregnant women and up to 29 per cent in pregnant women. Only a few antibiotics are able to redress this imbalance:

- Metronidazole – which frequently causes nausea and is poisonous in combination with alcohol. Metronidazole is best avoided or only used with caution during pregnancy.
- Co-amoxyclav – a penicillin combination drug which is also only used with caution during pregnancy.
- Clindamycin – usually given as a topical cream. This can be used with caution in pregnant women after the first three months of pregnancy.

Anaerobic vaginosis is best identified and treated early on in your pre-conceptual care programme. A recent study showed that women with bacterial vaginosis during the first sixteen weeks of pregnancy had more than five times the risk of miscarriage or pre-term labour than those with a normal vaginal balance.

Interestingly, the use of spermicidal contraceptive agents can halve the incidence of bacterial vaginosis, probably through killing anaerobic bacteria as well as sperm. In one study, 31 per cent of women not using spermicides had bacterial vaginosis compared with only 15 per cent of those using spermicidal preparations. Vaginal discharge and inflammation were also reduced (29 per cent compared with 44 per cent).

Chlamydia

Chlamydia trachomatis is one of the most common sexually transmissible diseases in the world. Through its ability to inflame and scar the Fallopian tubes, it is also the commonest cause of subfertility and ectopic pregnancy.

It is estimated that 10 per cent or more of the sexually active female population between the ages of 15 and 44 are infected, most without developing any early warning symptoms. Sometimes a discharge is noted; often there are no signs until pelvic inflammation causes pain. Infection is often picked up when their sexual partners develop a burning penile discharge.

Chlamydia are a strange cross between a bacterium and a virus. They are too small to be seen under the light microscope and are detected through special immunological laboratory tests. Swabs are taken from the cervix and urethra but results are not usually available for several days. If this infection is suspected, for example from a visible inflammation of the cervix or a pus-stained discharge, you will be given antibiotic treatment before the results are through. It is better to treat for chlamydia when you haven't got it than not to treat it when you have.

Chlamydia causes an ascending infection of the female genital tract. After a variable length of time, it reaches the Fallopian tubes to cause infection, inflammation and increasing amounts of scar tissue. This condition is known as pelvic inflammatory disease (PID) – see below.

If chlamydia infection is present during pregnancy, there is an increased risk of miscarriage and pre-term delivery. The baby is likely to pick up the infection during childbirth, developing sticky eyes (conjunctivitis), middle ear infection, genital infection or pneumonia. In many cases, this is the first sign that the mother is infected.

Pelvic inflammatory disease (PID)

PID is caused by chlamydia infection (plus anaerobic bacteria) in 70 per cent of cases. Infection is occasionally caused by gonorrhoea (10 per cent) or ascends after a surgical procedure such as termination of pregnancy or implantation of a coil.

It's estimated that 15 per cent of women have had symptomatic PID by the age of 30. After one attack of PID, 80 per cent of sufferers experience heavy or irregular periods and 40 per cent suffer deep pain during sexual intercourse. A further 20 per cent will experience chronic pelvic pain and 13 per cent will have difficulty conceiving as a result.

The risk of ectopic pregnancy (implantation of a fertilised egg somewhere other than the womb, e.g. in a Fallopian tube) is seven times greater in women who have had one attack of PID.

After a second attack of pelvic inflammatory disease, infertility rates rise to 35 per cent. After a third episode, 75 per cent of women are infertile because of scarring and blockage of the Fallopian tubes.

Inflammation and scarring results in poor penetration of antibiotics into the sites where infection lurks. Treatment therefore
consists of at least fourteen days' therapy with two or even three
different antibiotics.

Sexual partners should always be treated epidemiologically, or
on an 'in case' basis as studies suggest they are likely to be infected.
This prevents possible re-infection once you have recovered and
resumed an active sex life.

Genital herpes

Genital infection with the herpes simplex virus (HSV) causes a
spectrum of clinical illness. This ranges from symptomless viral
shedding to a severe 'flu-like illness with extensive genital
ulceration.

Up to 60 per cent of the population show evidence of previous
infection with HSV. Genital herpes forms two distinct patterns of
disease, each of which has different implications during pregnancy:

• The primary attack – when someone is exposed to genital
  herpes for the first time.
• Recurrent attacks when the person suffers a relapse.

The first (primary) attack of HSV infection usually lasts up to
fourteen days. The classic herpetic lesion starts as a red, inflamed
lump which breaks down to form a blister (vesicle) and then an
oval-shaped ulcer. These ulcers weep a watery, pus-stained fluid
which is highly infectious. In 80 per cent of women, the cervix is
ulcerated and secretes a copious discharge too. Lesions heal after
another seven to 10 days so the entire duration of the illness is
about three weeks. Viral shedding lasts up to 11 days. During this
first attack, viral particles travel up local nerve endings and lie
dormant in nerve ganglia near the spinal cord.

In half of all sufferers, the virus periodically reactivates and
travels down the nerve to cause a recurrent infection. Recurrent
infections are usually much milder than the primary attack and
ulcers tend to last for only three to four days.

Several factors are known to trigger recurrences of latent genital herpes infection. These include:

- Physical or mental stress.
- Menstruation.
- Pregnancy.
- Exposure to ultra-violet light.
- General ill health, especially other viral infections.
- Excessive heat or cold.
- Local genital trauma, e.g. rough sexual intercourse.
- Immunosuppressive drugs (e.g. corticosteriods).

Herpes simplex infection during pregnancy

A *primary* genital HSV infection during early pregnancy may result in miscarriage. The risk has been estimated at 25 per cent – but this is almost certainly an over-estimate. Other studies suggest that spreading of the virus across the placenta to the foetus is rare.

Primary HSV infection during the first three months of pregnancy may rarely produce foetal abnormalities which include:

- Skin lesions.
- Abnormally small eyes (microphthalmia).
- Inflammation at the back of the eye (chorioretinitis).
- Small head (microcephaly).

The risk to the foetus is small and primary infection is not considered an indication for therapeutic termination.

Recurrent attacks tend to be more common during the last three months of pregnancy than during the first six months. Fortunately, recurrent HSV attacks pose negligible risk to the foetus, except during delivery.

As the mother already has circulating anti-herpes antibodies (produced during the primary attack) her baby is protected. Recurrent attacks remain localised and do not spread across the placenta, unless there is a serious immunological abnormality.

If active genital herpes sores are present at the time of delivery, there is a small chance (5 to 10 per cent) that the baby could acquire infection during birth. Rarely, this might cause widespread infection such as viral meningitis or pneumonia. This is most likely to happen if the infection is a primary infection, however, as you will not have had time to develop any antibodies that might help to protect your baby. If a primary attack occurs at the time of delivery, a Caesarean is usually recommended. This is not routinely necessary for a recurrent attack as your baby will have protection from your own antibodies – however, it depends on the severity of the attack and the opinion of your obstetrician. The availability of antiviral drugs means that, on the few occasions in which a baby does become unwell, treatment with such drugs is very effective. If you are worried about this aspect of having had a herpes infection, it is important to discuss this with your obstetrician during pregnancy and to find out what his or her policy is on the subject.

Neonatal infection with genital herpes

The incidence of neonatal (newborn) herpes infection is increasing. In the USA, one case occurs per 5,000 live births. In the UK, the figure is much lower, at around one per 30,000 live births.

Unfortunately, up to 70 per cent of babies diagnosed as having neonatal herpes are born to mothers with no symptoms or signs at the time of delivery. Mothers with previous genital HVS infection are probably shedding virus asymptomatically at the time of delivery. Neonatal herpes is a serious illness causing:

- Skin vesicles (blisters) in 75 per cent of cases.
- Meningitis.
- Epileptic fits.
- Conjunctivitis.
- Breathing difficulties.
- Enlarged liver and spleen, with jaundice.

It is important that any woman who thinks (or knows) that she suffers from genital herpes should inform her obstetrician early on during her pregnancy – and should ideally seek advice during the pre-conceptual care period.

Genital warts

Genital warts are benign skin tumours caused by the human papilloma virus, of which over 50 types are known. Genital wart infection is so common some specialists consider it an epidemic.

Genital warts in women appear on the vulva or around the anus. Sufferers may have only one small, knobbly wart, several larger flat ones or numerous tiny, finger-like growths. In a few patients, especially during pregnancy, genital warts grow profusely to form a cauliflower-like lump the size of a golf ball!

If you think you have genital warts, it is important that these are treated during your pre-conceptual programme if possible. Once your hormonal status changes during pregnancy, they may start to grow rapidly and become more difficult to remove.

Genital warts can be treated in several ways. Those that are soft and non-keratinised are usually painted with a solution or cream containing podophyllotoxin which is the purified, active ingredient of the older podophyllin paint. Podophyllotoxin is a cytotoxic substance that literally kills wart-infected cells. Podophyllotoxin is increasingly used as a home-based treatment in which you apply the dilute solution or cream twice daily for three days per week over a maximum of five weeks before being re-assessed. Podophyllotoxin and podophyllin must not be used during pregnancy, as they may be absorbed to cause developmental abnormalities.

Podophyllotoxin is painted on at weekly intervals. This usually takes months to produce a satisfactory result. Podophyllotoxin must not be used during pregnancy as it is a potent cause of foetal abnormality. Adequate contraception should be used during and for four weeks after its use. It is not an ideal wart treatment during the pre-conceptual period.

Trichloro-acetic acid (TCA) is a strong acid that instantly coagulates a wart. Usually only a few treatments are needed to frighten lesions away. TCA and podophyllotoxin may be used together for more rapid results so long as pregnancy is excluded. TCA alone may be used to treat small genital warts during pregnancy itself. If too much TCA is applied, small chemical burns may result which take several days to heal.

Genital warts may also be frozen using a special probe. Regular repeat sessions are usually needed before the warts disappear. Cryotherapy may be used during pregnancy.

Electrocautery using a special bipolar electrical machine is another option. This equipment is expensive and not every genito-urinary unit has one. Warts are numbed with a local anaesthetic injection and then grasped between a pair of forceps connected to the machine. A blast of cauterising bipolar electricity is passed through the wart, which is literally vaporised. The shallow burn heals over the following week and results are instant and gratifying. This is an excellent method for treating the larger genital warts that can occur during pregnancy.

The latest treatment for genital warts is imiquimod, a drug that stimulates the body's own immune system to attack the viruses that cause genital warts. It is therefore known as an immune response modifier. Unlike podophyllotoxin, it does not have any antiviral action itself. Imiquimod cream is applied three times a week to the wart area before you go to sleep and is then washed off six to 10 hours later (e.g. next morning) with mild soap and water. While the cream is in place, you should avoid showering, bathing or sexual contact. Treatment continues until the warts clear or for a maximum of 16 weeks. It seems to be effective, with 72 per cent of users experiencing total clearance of warts. Recurrence rates are also low with imiquimod at 13 per cent compared with up to 65% with podophyllin alone, up to 34 per cent with podophyllotoxin and up to 39 per cent with cryotherapy. Side effects include local skin reactions such as redness, soreness, flaking and swelling. Treatment is only available on prescription and may be reserved until other, cheaper treatments have failed. It should not be used if pregnancy is suspected.

Gonorrhoea

Gonorrhoea is a sexually transmissible disease caused by neisseria gonorrhoea.

Infection in women may pass unnoticed, although sometimes an increased, pus-stained discharge occurs. Once diagnosed, infection is easily treated with a single dose of the new antibiotic ciprofloxacin, or with a penicillin combination. Undiagnosed infection may ascend into the Fallopian tubes to cause pelvic inflammatory disease (see page 137).

Syphilis

Despite blood screening for syphilis during pregnancy, between 50 and 60 children are still found to have congenital syphilis each year.

Syphilis is a sexually transmissible disease caused by the bacterium treponema pallidum. Within hours of infection, the motile bacteria enter the bloodstream and spread all over the body.

Three to four weeks later a painless, shallow ulcer (chancre) forms at the site of the infection – usually the genitals. This ulcer is highly infectious and is known as the primary sore. It heals after one to two months and usually leaves a faint scar.

Six to eight weeks after infection, some sufferers experience a mild 'flu-like illness and skin rash. The hair may fall out in clumps and large, flat wart-like growths may appear on the genitals. Many infected people don't develop these symptoms but are still infectious in this secondary stage of the disease.

If left untreated, syphilis causes problems again around ten years later – so-called tertiary syphilis. Tissue destruction occurs at variable sites, the heart and aorta (main artery) may become weakened or a form of madness (neurosyphilis) occurs which leads to paralysis.

If a mother has untreated syphilis, there is:

- A 33 per cent chance that her baby will be born healthy.
- A 33 per cent chance that the pregnancy will end in miscarriage or stillbirth.
- A 33 per cent chance that a live baby will have congenital syphilis syndrome.

Congenital syphilis causes foetal abnormalities such as:

- A flat, shrivelled face.
- A deformed, saddle-shaped nose.

- Wide-spaced, notched, peg-like teeth.
- Mental retardation.
- Skin rash with pock marks.
- Enlarged liver and spleen, possibly with jaundice.
- Future eye and joint problems.

Syphilis is routinely tested for by a blood test taken at ten to twelve weeks of pregnancy during the first antenatal visit. Ideally, pre-conceptual testing for syphilis is better as the disease can cross the placenta during early pregnancy to affect foetal development. If diagnosed, treatment is with antibiotics such as penicillin.

HIV and AIDS

The human immuno-deficiency virus (HIV) invades a type of white blood cell known as CD4 (helper) lymphocytes. These cells are vital in mobilising the body's defences to fight infection. To begin with, HIV lies dormant although some people experience a short-lived illness similar to glandular fever. This acute illness occurs two to six weeks after infection and consists of fever, sore throat, lethargy and joint pain. Glands (lymph nodes) may be enlarged. Sometimes a non-specific viral rash occurs on the trunk and upper limbs.

Only a high index of suspicion is likely to lead to an early diagnosis. For some reason, this early stage is more commonly reported in Australia than in the UK.

Two to three months after infection, the body mounts a weak antibody attack against the viral invader. In most cases, this is not enough to clear the infection. But these antibodies are a useful sign that a person has been exposed to HIV infection. If these antibodies are found on special blood (or saliva) testing, the person is said to be HIV (antibody) positive.

People who are HIV positive may remain well for many years. Some develop vague symptoms such as weight loss, fevers, sweats or unexplained diarrhoea.

If HIV is active, it invades and kills increasing numbers of CD4 cells. The ability of the immune system to fight infection falls and sufferers become prey to a number of exotic illnesses that normally do not trouble healthy humans. This stage of the disease is known as Acquired Immuno Deficiency Syndrome – AIDS for short.

How is HIV passed on?

HIV is passed on through intimate contact with infected blood, semen, vaginal fluids or breast milk. There are three main ways to catch it:

- Through unprotected sex (anal or vaginal) with an infected person (male or female).
- Through contact with infected blood (e.g. drug users sharing contaminated needles; transfusions).
- Infection from mother to baby in the womb or through breast feeding.

HIV is routinely tested for during pregnancy but only with your permission after counselling.

Specialists are urging pregnant women to have a voluntary HIV test. This is so that a mother who knows she is HIV positive can help prevent passing on the virus to her baby by avoiding breast feeding. The risk of an HIV positive woman passing the virus on to her baby if she does not breast feed is 15 per cent. Breast feeding increases this risk to 30 per cent.

If you are HIV positive and want to have a baby, other steps can be taken to reduce the risk of passing infection to the baby. You will be advised to time your pregnancy after treatment to ensure your CD4 cell count is high, and the viral load (amount of virus in your blood) is low, as this has been shown to reduce the chances of exposing the baby to the virus. The use of antiviral drugs during pregnancy and delivery can reduce the risk of transmission of HIV from the mother to the baby by two thirds. Having a Caesarean also helps to protect the baby.

Safer sex

Our main protection against HIV and other sexually transmissible diseases is through safer sex. Strong condoms and/or dental dams (squares of latex placed over female genitalia during oral sex) should always be used where appropriate. It is important to remember that sex, even safer sex, with at-risk partners (e.g. bisexuals, drug abusers, casual contacts abroad or with those from endemic countries) greatly increases your chances of contracting HIV.

Women who have successfully conceived, but whose circumstances place them at risk of contracting a sexually transmissible disease during pregnancy, are advised to continue using condoms during sex. Even though the need for contraception is gone, condoms can provide some protection for both mother and child against most genito-urinary infections.

12

Other harmful infections

This chapter concentrates on other infections that can cause problems if contracted just before or during pregnancy.

Listeria

Listeriosis is a bacterial infection that is common in cattle, pigs and poultry and which is also widespread in the soil. It can infect humans, causing a 'flu-like illness up to six weeks after exposure.

The disease is life-threatening in the elderly, those with poor immunity, in pregnant women and in the newborn baby. Listeria can be passed from mother to child at any stage during pregnancy, but infection remains relatively rare at around one case per 30,000 births. Listeria infection during pregnancy is linked with miscarriage, stillbirth, pre-term delivery and severe illness in the newborn (e.g. meningitis, pneumonia).

Foods with a high listeria risk should be avoided throughout the pre-conceptual period and during pregnancy itself (see also page 56). The bacterium is usually destroyed by pasteurisation but if food is infected and then refrigerated, listeria continues to multiply. Avoid foods such as:

- Ripened soft cheeses, e.g. Brie, Camembert, Cambozola.
- Blue-veined cheeses, e.g. Stilton, Roquefort, blue Shropshire, blue Brie, Dolcelatte.
- Goat or sheep cheeses, e.g. feta, chèvres.
- Any unpasteurised soft and cream cheese.

- Undercooked meat.
- Cook-chill meals and ready-to-eat poultry unless thoroughly reheated.
- All types of pâté.
- Ready-prepared coleslaw and salads.
- Unpasteurised milk or dairy products.
- All foods past their 'best by' date.
- Rolls and sandwiches containing any of the above.

All hard Cheddar-type cheeses are safe, as are cottage cheese, soft processed cheese spreads and cream cheese.

Listeria can also be passed on through contact with infected live animals.

Women who are contemplating pregnancy should be especially careful to follow the above guidelines when travelling abroad. The incidence of food contamination and infection is high in many countries.

Treatment of suspected listeriosis cases is with hospitalisation and high-dose antibiotics.

Toxoplasmosis

Toxoplasmosis is an infection caused by a single-celled organism (protozoan). It can be caught from eating raw or undercooked meat, unwashed fruit and vegetables, drinking unpasteurised milk, or from handling cats' faeces.

It is estimated that 25 per cent of pork and 10 per cent of lamb eaten by humans is infected, but cysts are killed by thorough cooking and by freezing. Toxoplasma also multiplies in cats and around 1 per cent of cats excrete toxoplasma eggs in their faeces.

Infection is not dangerous to the healthy adult or child. Symptoms of human infection may be similar to mild 'flu or glandular fever, but often pass unnoticed. Only around 700 cases are recognised annually in the UK.

Toxoplasma is an important organism because if contracted during pregnancy, it is associated with miscarriage, stillbirth and/or foetal abnormalities. These include:

- Hydrocephalus.
- Eye defects and blindness.
- Physical and mental retardation.
- Convulsions.
- Small head (microcephaly).
- Calcification of parts of the brain.
- Enlarged liver and spleen.
- Increased risk of death during infancy.

During the second half of pregnancy, damage to the foetus is less severe.

Research suggests that only 15 per cent of antenatal women are immune, implying that 85 per cent of pregnant women are at risk of infection. It's estimated that between two and five women out of every 1,000 contract toxoplasmosis during pregnancy.

Some researchers estimate that an infected pregnant woman has a 30 per cent to 40 per cent chance of passing the infection on to her baby, with a 10 per cent chance that the foetus will be severely affected. Studies of the prevalence of disease suggest the risks are four times lower than this as only around 12 severely damaged babies are born each year.

Toxoplasmosis can only be ruled out by a series of blood tests taken throughout pregnancy and during the first year of a child's life. No single test can assure you that your baby is not at risk. Treatment is usually with the anti-malarial drug pyrimethamine and a sulphonamide antibiotic.

Experts claim that 70 per cent of women with acute toxoplasmosis during pregnancy are not followed up properly. Their babies, even though asymptomatic at birth, may still be infected and, unless treated, may suffer irreversible damage with future learning difficulties. This is obviously quite worrying.

Testing for toxoplasmosis

- Any screening must involve repeated blood tests throughout pregnancy.
- Testing can result in false positives and false negatives.

- When infection is suspected, foetal blood sampling can help detect the presence of parasites or foetal antibodies.
- Many affected babies are born without symptoms and, if not treated, will suffer damage over the next year.
- It is not known whether testing does more harm than good, in raising levels of anxiety.

All women who are contemplating pregnancy or who are pregnant are strongly advised to follow the simple precautions outlined below.

How to protect yourself from toxoplasmosis during pre-conceptual care and throughout pregnancy

- Avoid emptying cat litter trays.
- If having to handle cat litter, use thick, disposable gloves and wash your hands thoroughly afterwards with an antiseptic solution.
- Always wash hands thoroughly after handling cats.
- Avoid close contact with sick cats.
- Always wash your hands well after contact with earth or animals.
- Avoid eating raw meat or fish and their products.
- Wash hands thoroughly after handling raw meat.
- Cook all meat thoroughly, wash fruit and vegetables and avoid unpasteurised milk – especially goats' milk and products.
- Freezing kills the reproductive cysts of toxoplasmosis. It may be worth pregnant women eating more frozen meat.
- Sheep and lambs are a source of toxoplasma as well as other organisms associated with recurrent miscarriage (chlamydia psittaci). Women who are contemplating pregnancy, or already pregnant, should avoid contact with sheep, especially pregnant or milking ewes and newborn lambs. It is especially important to avoid contact with aborted lambs and with all placentas. If you do develop a fever or 'flu-like symptoms after being in contact with sheep, seek medical advice immediately.

Chickenpox

If chickenpox is contracted during the first three months of pregnancy, there is a 3 per cent risk of it causing foetal abnormalities known as Varicella Syndrome. Maternal infection from four months' pregnancy onwards seems to cause no problems unless it is at delivery.

Foetal abnormalities are similar to those found in Rubella Syndrome, including:

- Cataracts and other eye defects, blindness.
- Small head (microcephaly).
- Excess cerebro-spinal fluid (hydrocephaly).
- Skin pock marks.

Unlike Rubella Syndrome, the foetus does not continue to shed infectious viral particles after birth.

If the mother contracts chickenpox just before or after delivery, the foetus may contract a severe form of the disease with viral meningitis and pneumonia. The mortality rate is then in the region of 30 per cent.

Avoid anyone who has chickenpox or shingles throughout the pre-conceptual period and pregnancy. Shingles is caused by reactivation of dormant chickenpox virus and causes a patch of highly infectious blisters on the skin. It is possible to catch chickenpox (but not shingles) from these.

If you do come into contact with a person who has chickenpox or shingles during the pre-conceptual care period or during pregnancy, seek medical help straight away. An injection of anti-varicella zoster immunoglobulin (antibodies) will help protect both you and your future child.

Some public health doctors believe that pregnant women should be routinely screened for immunity to chickenpox and given immunoglobulin if they are found vulnerable to infection. Varicella vaccines are available in some parts of the world. As soon as they become available in the UK, routine pre-conceptual screening is likely to start in a similar manner to that for rubella.

Cytomegalovirus (CMV)

Cytomegalovirus belongs to the same family of viruses as those causing genital herpes, chickenpox and shingles. Infection with CMV is common and antibodies in around 80 per cent of adults suggest previous exposure to the disease. CMV may cause a mild 'flu-like illness but in many cases infection passes unnoticed.

This is another example of an infection that can be passed from mother to child during pregnancy with devastating results. The earlier in pregnancy that infection occurs, the more severe the outcome. Infection is linked with:

- Miscarriage and pre-term labour.
- Small head.
- Physical and mental retardation.
- Developmental difficulties.
- Progressive hearing problems.
- Jaundice.
- Intra-uterine growth retardation.
- Chest and eye infections.

It is estimated that 3,000 babies are infected per year, with 300 suffering a subsequent handicap.

There are no obvious protective measures to take, except for avoiding animals or humans who are clearly sick.

Vaccinations

Women who are in the pre-conceptual care period or already pregnant should avoid immunisation with any vaccines containing live viruses. These viruses have been changed (attenuated) so they are no longer capable of causing serious disease. However, they still multiply within the body to confer immunity. Occasionally, attenuated viruses revert to the wild (pathogenic) type and can cause a mild version of the illness against which vaccination was given.

Adequate contraception should always be used during immunisation with live vaccine and for one month afterwards. Live vaccines are only administered during pregnancy when the benefits are thought to outweigh the risks.

Immunisation with vaccines containing killed (inactivated) micro-organisms, or toxins, offers little risk to the foetus. But like all other vaccines, it should generally be avoided during pregnancy unless there is a definite risk of infection.

When due to have an immunisation, always tell your doctor if you are thinking about having a baby. You may be advised to use adequate contraception during vaccination and for one month afterwards. If you are already pregnant, you may be advised to wait until the pregnancy is over before receiving certain injections.

If the benefits of vaccination outweigh the risks of infection, you may be advised to have the injection – but make sure you know all the pros and cons before making a decision to go ahead.

13

Smoking, alcohol and drugs

Smoking – females

Smoking is one of the major causes of preventable disease and early death in the Western world. On average, it cuts six years off the life of a moderate smoker.

Smoking during the pre-conceptual care period and pregnancy is especially harmful as it affects your ability to rear healthy children in the following ways:

- Subfertility is three times more common in smokers.
- Smoking mothers have a 27 per cent higher chance of a miscarriage than non-smokers.
- Passive smoking is involved in 4,000 miscarriages per year.
- Smoking during pregnancy causes malfunction of the placenta, stillbirth, low-birth-weight babies and babies of lower intelligence.
- Babies born to smoking mothers are on average 200 g lighter than babies born to non-smokers.
- Babies born to smoking mothers have a 28 per cent higher risk of death around the time of birth than babies born to non-smokers.
- Estimates in the US suggest that eliminating smoking in pregnancy could prevent 5 per cent of foetal and neonatal deaths, 20 per cent of low-birth-weight babies and 8 per cent of pre-term deliveries.

- Up to a quarter of all cot deaths are associated with passive smoking.
- Women who smoke during pregnancy increase by a third the risk of the child developing asthma.
- Mothers who smoke during pregnancy are twice as likely to have children with behavioural problems – possibly due to foetal brain damage during development.
- Passive smoking causes asthma, chest infections, eczema and glue ear in young children.
- There are 4,000 different chemicals present in tobacco smoke of which many are carcinogenic (cancer forming). Exposure to chemicals from a smoking mother (or father) increases the risk of a foetus later developing childhood cancer (see page 157).

Smoking and decreased female fertility

Many studies have shown a link between female smokers and sub-fertility. One study showed that 38 per cent of non-smokers conceived during their first menstrual cycle after stopping contraception compared to only 28 per cent of smokers.

Another study showed that twice as many females smoking ten or more cigarettes per day remained involuntarily childless after five years (10.7 per cent) compared to non-smoking women (5.4 per cent).

A similar relationship holds true for women undergoing assisted fertilisation techniques. In one trial, 72 per cent of eggs collected from non-smoking women were successfully fertilised in a test tube compared to only 44 per cent of eggs collected from smoking women. This difference in egg receptivity is critical when the partner's sperm also have a low natural fertilising capacity – perhaps also due to smoking (see page 215).

Whether or not smoking is the actual cause of female subfertility cannot be proved until a definite, measurable mechanism is identified. Several theories have been suggested:

- Women smokers have lower circulating oestrogen hormone levels, which may affect egg maturation.
- Nicotine and arabinase (two components of cigarette smoke) are known to inhibit an ovarian enzyme which helps to convert

steroid hormones into oestrogen – one reason why smokers' oestrogen levels are low.

- Nicotine and its metabolite, conitine, also inhibit another enzyme which is needed for the production of oestrogen hormone.
- Nicotine has several effects on the egg which are similar to natural events preventing more than one sperm entering the egg (cortical granule formation). These nicotine effects may stop even one sperm from entering the egg.
- Nicotine is concentrated in the dividing fertilised egg (blastocyst) and may have a direct effect on implantation and early embryonic development.
- Smoking is linked with a woman entering the menopause one to two years earlier than non-smokers – there's evidence that passive smoking hastens the menopause too.

All women who are hoping to have a baby should stop smoking before attempting to conceive for both their own and their future child's health.

Exposure of the developing foetus to tobacco smoke

From the moment of conception, all embryos – but especially those of smoking mothers – are exposed to nicotine and tobacco. Biochemical measurements confirm that constituents of cigarette smoke are found in the placenta, amniotic fluid and foetal blood of both actively and passively smoking mothers. All babies are therefore exposed to cigarettes before birth.

In the UK, 28 per cent of mothers smoke during pregnancy. In the USA, 31 per cent of married mothers smoked before conceiving and 26 per cent continued to smoke during pregnancy. Only 5 per cent managed to give up.

Even if you don't smoke yourself, the risk to your baby is increased if someone else in your household does. Passive smoking of at least one hour per week has been reported for 63 per cent of non-smoking adults. This figure will hopefully drop as smoking in public becomes less widely acceptable.

Effects of exposure to cigarette smoke during gestation

Every time a smoking mother puffs a cigarette, the nicotine she absorbs causes spasm and narrowing of important arteries. This spasm also occurs in vessels within the uterus and placenta.

By narrowing arteries which supply blood to the placenta and developing embryo, smoking decreases the amount of oxygen and nourishment they receive. This is one reason why smokers tend to give birth to smaller babies than non-smokers. Another reason for growth retardation is that smoking generates carbon monoxide – a molecule that displaces oxygen from haemoglobin in red blood cells. These two factors combined mean that less blood, which is less rich in oxygen, is supplied to the baby.

Stopping smoking at any stage of pregnancy is better than continuing to smoke all the way through – it is never too late to improve your baby's health.

In one study, 800 smokers were followed throughout pregnancy with their tobacco consumption accurately measured. Mothers who quit smoking during the pregnancy gave birth to infants that were an average of 241 g heavier than babies born to mothers who continued to smoke and 167 g heavier than babies born to mothers who managed to cut back. Babies born to those who cut back were 74 g heavier than babies born to those continuing to smoke – so benefit is gained even if a mother finds it impossible to give up completely.

Pre-conceptual exposure to tobacco smoke and the subsequent development of childhood cancer

Apart from the effects on the baby's growth and potential intelligence, researchers estimate that 6 per cent of all childhood cancers and 17 per cent of acute lymphocytic leukaemias are associated with maternal smoking during the pre-conceptual care period and the first three months of pregnancy. Independent studies show strong associations between maternal smoking and the child later developing:

- Leukaemia – with a two-fold increased risk of acute lymphocytic leukaemia.
- Non-Hodgkin's lymphoma (a cancer of the lymphatic system) – two-fold increased risk.
- Wilm's tumour (a type of kidney cancer) – two-fold increased risk.
- Brain cancer.

Risks are even greater if the father smokes during the twelve months prior to the child's birth (see page 215).

A study performed by the National Institute of Environmental Health, North Carolina, USA, looked at 220 children under the age of fourteen suffering from cancer. They calculated the increased risk of childhood cancers in children whose mothers smoked during the pre-conceptual care period (i.e. three months prior to conception), continued to smoke during the first three months of pregnancy and then gave up or smoked throughout the entire pregnancy.

Overall, when mothers smoked during the three months prior to conception, children had a 30 per cent higher risk of developing a childhood cancer compared to children whose mothers did not smoke. The risk of acute lymphocytic leukaemia or lymphoma was twice as high.

For children whose mothers continued to smoke during the first three months of pregnancy, their overall increased risk of developing cancer was 50 per cent higher than children whose mothers did not smoke.

When both mothers and fathers smoked, the odds rose to an overall 50 per cent greater risk of the child later developing any type of cancer, with the risks of acute lymphatic leukaemia and lymphomas more than doubled.

As parents who smoke throughout the time the mother is pregnant tend to continue smoking throughout the baby's early years, the child continues to be exposed.

For all the reasons outlined above, it is vital to stop smoking before the pre-conceptual care period. If you are currently smoking and thinking of having a baby, review the facts and decide which is the healthiest option for you and your child. Maternal smoking is among the most common potentially harmful exposures a baby will encounter during development – and it is a major public health concern.

The ideal goal for smoking women is to give up smoking altogether – but cutting back is definitely better than nothing. You may find using a carbon monoxide monitor has a positive, reinforcing effect on your resolve.

A simple 'quit plan' is outlined below. Your doctor will be pleased to help you, too.

Stopping smoking

Nicotine is addictive, which is why it is so difficult to give up smoking. Withdrawal symptoms of tension, aggression, depression, insomnia and craving can occur.

The good news is that within 48 hours of giving up smoking, levels of clotting factors in the blood start to fall. This will reduce the risk of placental insufficiency, growth retardation and low birth weight of your future child.

A simple quit plan

- Name the day you're going to give up and get into the right frame of mind.
- Find support – giving up nicotine is easier with a friend or partner. If the potential father of your child smokes, it is essential that he stops too. You will find it easier giving up if you do it together.
- Get rid of temptation. Throw away all smoking paraphernalia – papers, matches, lighters, ashtrays, spare packets, etc.
- Find a hobby to take your mind off smoking. Try becoming more active – increase the amount of regular exercise you take to improve your overall fitness.
- Identify situations where you would usually smoke and either avoid them or plan ahead to overcome them.
- Watch your diet. Avoid excess saturated fats and count calories so you don't put on weight. Chew sugar-free gum or drink water and diet drinks instead.

- Take things one day at a time. Every morning, say to yourself, 'I just have to get through today.' If you think longer term, you're more likely to give in.
- Keep a star chart and stick on a gold star every day you last without a cigarette. Plan a reward for every week of success. Psychological tricks like this sound ridiculous – but they work.
- Learn to relax. Have a massage, practise yoga or meditation. You need something to replace the anxiety-relieving effects of nicotine.
- Save the money previously spent on cigarettes in a special fund. Buy a luxury for yourself – or save it to spend on your future baby.
- When the going gets tough, indulge in some positive thought. First, picture a growing baby in your mind, receiving its life blood through healthy vessels in the placenta. Now imagine these vessels constricting with every puff on a cigarette. See the blue, oxygen-poor blood supply to the baby slow down to a trickle and the baby's growth slow down. Now think positive again – see the arteries in the womb and placenta dilate, pumping oxygen-rich blood into your healthy, thriving baby.

Shock tactics – but you *must* give up to give your baby the best possible start in life that you can. It's in your hands.

Nicotine replacement therapy

If you find it difficult to quit smoking during your pre-conceptual care programme, consider using nicotine replacement products such as skin patches, chewing gum or spray. The quit rate with nicotine replacement patches or gum is double that of people going it alone. New research suggests that nicotine nasal sprays are three times more effective in helping people remain cigarette-free after one year.

Nicotine replacement must not be used during pregnancy, however. Stop using nicotine replacement at least six weeks before you start trying to conceive. Nicotine has adverse effects on fertility, on the fertilised egg and on the foetus.

Complementary therapy

Alternative medical techniques can also help you stop smoking. Hypnotherapy, acupuncture, flotation, aromatherapy and relaxation therapy have often succeeded where will-power has failed. Hypnotherapy has a success rate of 30 per cent – better even than using nicotine replacement patches.

Relaxation exercise

A useful relaxation exercise to alleviate your cravings for nicotine is as follows:

- Breathe in deeply through your mouth and feel your rib cage expand to its fullest capacity.
- Hold your breath for three seconds.
- Let out all the air slowly, until your lungs feel totally empty.
- Hold your breath for a further three seconds.
- Repeat this cycle twice more, so you have breathed in and out slowly a total of three times.
- Now breathe normally again.

Stopping smoking and pre-conceptual care

Once you are confident that you have succeeded in giving up smoking (e.g. at least six to eight weeks since your last cigarette) you should then ideally wait an additional three months before trying to conceive.

Throughout the time of initially stopping smoking until you start trying to conceive, follow your pre-conceptual care programme in earnest. This will give your baby the best possible start in life.

Alcohol, pre-conceptual care and pregnancy

Alcohol is the most widely available drug in the world. In the West, 90 per cent of adults indulge – even if only occasionally.

The recommended healthy limit for non-pregnant women is fourteen units per week but one in six women drink more than this. An estimated 200,000 women in the UK drink more than 35 units per week, which, on a regular basis, will seriously damage their health. More importantly, alcohol can seriously damage a developing baby. If a woman regularly drinks more than twelve units of alcohol per week during pregnancy, her baby will suffer growth retardation and birth weight will be lower than normal.

UK units

1 unit alcohol	= 100 ml (one glass) of wine
(8 g ethanol)	= 50 ml (one measure) of sherry
	= 25 ml (single tot) of spirit
	= 300 ml (1/2 pint) of beer.

NB In the USA, a unit of alcohol is called a 'drink'.

In a study involving 321 pregnant women, the difference in size (millilitres) between self-selected drinks and standard-sized drinks was significant. Drinks that were self-poured were, on average, 49 per cent above the standard size (for beer), and up to 307 per cent above the standard size for spirits. For some women, their pre-pregnancy average alcohol intake was actually four to almost 10 times higher when self-defined drink sizes were taken into account. The researchers were concerned that, where women give birth to a baby with foetal alcohol syndrome, the relative risks per unit of alcohol may be higher than previously thought if they were based on underestimates of alcohol intake.

Alcohol and fertility

Alcohol also seems to affect the chance of conception. In a survey, 430 Danish couples aged 20–35 years who were trying to conceive for the first time were followed over six menstrual cycles or until pregnancy occurred. Average weekly alcohol intake was 4.0 drinks among the women and 9.5 drinks among their male partners. Only 17 per cent abstained from alcohol throughout the six cycles in which they were followed. The researchers found that a woman's alcohol intake was linked with decreased fertility, even among women with a weekly alcohol intake corresponding to five or fewer drinks. In the six cycles of follow-up, 64 per cent of women with a weekly alcohol intake of less than five drinks and 55 per cent of women with a higher intake conceived. After taking into account other factors such as smoking, length of menstrual cycle, gynaecological conditions, weight and partner's sperm count, the chance of pregnancy was found to decrease with increasing alcohol intake from 61 per cent among women who had one to five drinks a week, to 55 per cent among those reporting six to 10 drinks a week down to 34 per cent for women consuming more than 10 drinks a week, compared with women not drinking any alcohol.

In one survey, half of women reported consuming alcohol during the three months before finding out they were pregnant, with one in 20 consuming six or more drinks per week. Of those who drank alcohol, 60 per cent did not learn they were pregnant until after the fourth week of gestation, and many did not know until after the sixth week. It therefore seems a good idea to avoid alcohol altogether when trying to become pregnant.

Women, alcohol and pregnancy

Women have a lower alcohol tolerance than men as we have twice as much fat – around 30 per cent of body weight compared to the male's more usual 15 per cent. Fatty tissue absorbs alcohol like a sponge and slowly releases it into the circulation. So alcohol stays in the female body longer than it does in the male's and is only slowly transported to the liver for metabolism.

Pregnancy is a time of massive physiological changes. Body fat stores increase by 10 per cent (variable) and blood volume goes up by about a third. This dilutes the effects of alcohol so a pregnant woman may subconsciously drink more than she did before pregnancy to achieve the same results.

For various reasons, mainly to do with the way alcohol is distributed through body fluids, the developing foetus receives a relatively higher blood concentration of alcohol than its mother. Alcohol also stays in foetal tissues longer, because the developing liver is less efficient at breaking it down. The tiny liver bud only develops during the fourth week after conception. So the time when the foetus is most vulnerable to alcohol damage – when it can't metabolise alcohol in self-defence – is the first month after conception. This is usually before the mother even knows she is pregnant.

Unless you take positive steps to avoid alcohol during the pre-conceptual period, you are at risk of harming your baby.

The cellular effects of alcohol

Alcohol is rapidly absorbed from the stomach and the first part of the intestines. It is broken down in the liver to form acetaldehyde, acetic acid and finally carbon dioxide and water.

Alcohol and its products of metabolism readily pass from the maternal bloodstream into the placenta and foetal circulation. These are poorly deactivated by the tiny foetal liver, once it is formed at four to seven weeks' gestation. A large maternal intake of alcohol, especially amounts due to binge drinking, can have serious consequences for the developing foetus.

Alcohol interferes with the action of almost every vitamin and many minerals. In particular, a woman who regularly drinks more than the safe weekly limit of alcohol is at risk of deficiency of vitamins B1, B2, B3, B6, folate, essential fatty acids, calcium, magnesium and zinc. This can have dire consequences for the foetus (see vitamins and minerals on pages 59–100).

Alcohol and miscarriage

There is an increased risk of a spontaneous abortion (miscarriage) in women who regularly drink even small amounts of alcohol. This is especially noticeable during the fourth to sixth months of pregnancy.

Miscarriage may be due to a direct effect of alcohol or its breakdown product, acetaldehyde. As researchers are not sure which is more likely, it is important that pregnant women avoid alcohol altogether.

If you do indulge during pregnancy, it is equally important to avoid drugs which interfere with alcohol metabolism and allow acetaldehyde to build up. The most frequently used drug with this effect is the antibiotic metronidazole. This is commonly prescribed for vaginal anaerobic bacterial infections (see page 135) and pelvic inflammatory disease (see page 137). Another such drug is disulfiram (Antabuse), which is used in the treatment of alcohol addiction.

Excessive alcohol intake increases the concentration of acids in maternal and foetal blood – a condition known as metabolic acidosis. This also affects foetal development and may trigger a miscarriage.

Alcohol affects cell membranes by damping their ability to conduct small electrical charges. This is exactly how general anaesthetics work and, in fact, alcohol is a weak general anaesthetic. In adults, this depressant action on brain cells causes drowsiness, stupor and, in excess, coma or even death. In the foetus it interferes with cellular communication and may trigger developmental abnormalities or miscarriage.

It's safest for a woman planning to have a baby to refrain from alcohol altogether during the pre-conceptual care period. Try to abstain for at least three months (preferably six) before conceiving until the baby is born.

Foetal Alcohol Syndrome

At the turn of the century, doctors noticed that 'inebriate mothers' were likely to produce offspring that were stillborn or died in early infancy. Those who survived were of low birth weight, unintelligent and displayed developmental difficulties. It wasn't until 1973 that these problems were labelled Foetal Alcohol Syndrome. This is a serious condition characterised by:

- A high risk of spontaneous abortion (miscarriage).
- A high risk of stillbirth.
- Low birth weight.
- Narrow, receding forehead.
- Short, upturned nose.
- Receding chin.
- Asymmetrical, poorly formed ears.
- Thin lips.

- Long distance between nose and lips, with flattened or absent skin folds.
- Short-sightedness (myopia).
- Squint (strabismus).
- Heavy folds (epicanthic) between the nose and eyes.
- Slanted eyes.
- Congenital heart disease.
- Low intelligence.

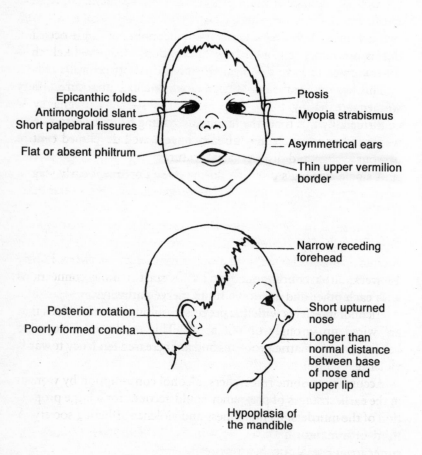

Epicanthic folds

Antimongoloid slant
Short palpebral fissures

Flat or absent philtrum

Ptosis

Myopia strabismus

Asymmetrical ears

Thin upper vermilion border

Narrow receding forehead

Posterior rotation
Poorly formed concha

Short upturned nose

Longer than normal distance between base of nose and upper lip

Hypoplasia of the mandible

Features of the Foetal Alcohol Syndrome

If a woman regularly drinks two or three units per day throughout pregnancy, she has an 11 per cent chance of her baby developing Foetal Alcohol Syndrome. This risk rises to 19 per cent with four units per day and to 30 per cent in women who drink more than five units daily.

A pregnant woman who regularly drinks more than nine units of alcohol per day is almost certain to have an affected child.

Isolated binge drinking

As well as regular drinking, maternal binge drinking is equally harmful to a developing foetus. A study of 1,008 women showed that a woman who drank ten units of alcohol on a single occasion during pregnancy (e.g. a birthday celebration) was more likely than other women to have a congenitally abnormal offspring.

This has important implications for pre-conceptual care. Many women are happy to give up alcohol as soon as pregnancy is confirmed. By this time, the foetus is anything from three to twelve weeks old or more. It may already have a well-developed central nervous system and distinct facial features.

A single evening's drinking during these important early stages, when a mother doesn't know she is pregnant, can affect your baby for life.

Alcohol and the foetal brain

A critical stage of foetal brain development occurs between 10 and 18 weeks after conception. Nerve cells start making connections with each other and lay down future nerve pathways.

Alcohol interferes with this process, resulting in connections that are wired up wrongly or not at all. This results in sociopathic behaviour, psychiatric problems and an increased tendency towards violence.

According to some researchers, alcohol consumption by women in the earliest stages of pregnancy could account for a large proportion of the murders, mental illness and violence afflicting society. A third of inmates on Death Row in the United States supposedly suffer from Foetal Alcohol Syndrome.

Isn't it now acceptable to have a little alcohol during pregnancy?

Recent studies suggest that low levels of maternal alcohol consumption (up to eight units spread throughout the week) are not linked with birth defects but confirm that heavy consumption is dangerous. The best advice is to avoid alcohol altogether in the pre-conception period (at least three months) and for the first three months of pregnancy. If you find it difficult to go without alcohol after this, the odd drink (one or two units) once or twice a week during the later stages of pregnancy is unlikely to do serious harm – but remember the increased risk of a spontaneous miscarriage.

Drugs

During the pre-conceptual care period, and throughout pregnancy, it is important to avoid taking all but the most essential of drugs.

Even aspirin and ibuprofen carry theoretical risks as they inhibit the production of certain hormone-like chemicals (prostaglandins) that are essential for reproduction and foetal development. They might also interfere with conception itself and affect fertility, especially if taken mid-cycle. Recent research has shown that taking a non-steroidal anti-inflammatory drug (e.g. ibuprofen) can increase the risk of miscarriage – especially if taken around the time of conception. Avoid all unnecessary drugs during the pre-conceptual period as well as during pregnancy.

As well as having a direct adverse effect on a developing foetus, many drugs also interfere with the absorption, action or excretion of vitamins and minerals. For example, alcohol increases the need for B vitamins, zinc and magnesium; some antibiotics antagonise the action of folate.

If you are taking prescribed drugs, inform your physician of your intention to try for a pregnancy. In some cases, medication will need to be changed to a (hopefully) safer treatment or withdrawn altogether.

Unfortunately, no drug can be assumed completely safe in any particular pregnancy as the tragic case of thalidomide has shown.

It is now thought that thalidomide caused its associated birth defects through precipitating a relative deficiency of vitamin B12.

Anticonvulsant drugs

Anticonvulsant drugs pose a dilemma in pregnancy. The mother must be prevented from having fits, but some anticonvulsants are associated with an increased risk of foetal abnormality. In most cases, this is caused by lowering folate levels by increasing the rate of its metabolism, and by increasing the requirements for vitamin D.

Although it seems logical to give additional folate supplements to epileptic women wishing to conceive, large amounts of folic acid antagonise the beneficial effects of anticonvulsant treatment and may lead to increased frequency of epileptic fits. A fine line must be drawn to balance drug dosage with nutrient intakes.

Always seek help

So many drugs are contraindicated in pregnancy – or should only be used under close medical supervision – that they cannot all be mentioned here.

In general, during the pre-conceptual care period and throughout pregnancy:

- Stop taking any over-the-counter drugs you have bought yourself, including antacids, sports gels, mild painkillers and illicit, recreational drugs.
- If you are taking any prescribed medication, discuss your intention to become pregnant with your prescribing doctor. You will be advised on which drugs you may safely continue taking and which ones should definitely be stopped or exchanged.

Cannabis

The hemp plant, cannabis sativa, is the source of cannabis resin and marijuana (the dried leaves and flower tops). Recreational use of these drugs is prohibited in many countries, but they remain widely available and widely used.

The active ingredient in cannabis and marijuana is tetra-hydrocannabinol (THC), a substance chemically related to steroid hormones such as oestrogen and progesterone. As a result, tetra-hydrocannabinol tends to accumulate in the ovaries.

Use of these recreational drugs can cause menstrual cycle irregularity in women. They also affect cell division and decrease the rate at which cells grow. Using cannabis or marijuana during pregnancy will affect foetal growth and result in low-birth-weight babies. There is some evidence that it prolongs or arrests labour, too.

Cocaine, crack and amphetamines

Cocaine and crack use among pregnant women significantly increases the risk of miscarriage or stillbirth and causes low-birth-weight babies.

Heroin

Heroin addiction leads to subfertility and increased complications during pregnancy. It is linked with a three times greater risk of miscarriage or stillbirth, a four times greater risk of premature labour and a significant risk of intra-uterine growth retardation. This results in low-birth-weight babies. The risks of congenital abnormalities and failure to thrive are also increased.

Babies born to addicted mothers are addicted too and have to go through their own, unpleasant process of withdrawal. This is associated with a 30 per cent risk of death in the perinatal period.

Women who inject drugs have an increased risk of blood poisoning (septicaemia), hepatitis B and HIV.

Overcoming drug addiction

Women who are addicted to recreational drugs, especially those as dangerous as heroin, are strongly advised to seek help to kick their habit before trying to conceive.

Drugs need to be slowly weaned off before pregnancy as withdrawal during pregnancy (especially if this is abrupt) can cause miscarriage or premature labour.

Detoxification programmes are now sophisticated, with a highly motivational and non-judgemental team approach.

14

Environmental and work-related toxins

The environment is full of toxins such as lead from exhaust fumes, mercury, industrial chemicals and pesticides. These enter the food chain and may contaminate a large percentage of our diet, whether we are vegetarians, fishitarians or omnivores.

Toxins build up and can trigger problems such as dietary allergy, skin diseases, asthma, other immunological disorders, infertility and even cancer. Most people, however, feel perfectly healthy despite potentially harmful levels inside them.

Over 30 years ago, the tragedy of thalidomide taught us that all chemicals and drugs should be tested for their potentially damaging effects – not just to those already born, but to the developing foetus as well – before being approved for widespread use. Since then, we've discovered that a wide range of drugs, pesticides, food additives and other industrial chemicals can cause birth defects, subfertility and abnormal development in children.

Unfortunately, of more than 60,000 man-made chemicals now in use, only 4,000 have been evaluated as to their effects on the process of human reproduction.

Most environmental toxins cross the placenta and pose a risk to the developing foetus. A study by the Women's Environmental Network suggests that up to 8 per cent of British children suffer from poor responsiveness and memory loss because of toxic damage in the womb. They may also have reduced intelligence in later life. Even if only 1 per cent are affected, this still represents thousands of children per year.

To avoid these risks, a potential mother and father should consider switching to a detoxifying diet during their pre-conceptual care programme. To protect the unborn child from neurological damage, dietary modifications need to start before conception.

This chapter looks briefly at some of the potentially hazardous environmental and workplace-related toxins we are likely to encounter. It includes simple tips on how to avoid excessive exposure.

Toxic heavy metals

Cadmium

Cadmium is a common pollutant linked with infertility and stillbirth, especially when coupled with high lead and low zinc levels. It is also associated with cleft palate, hare lip, low birth weight, small head and congenital limb abnormalities. Our main sources of cadmium are from:

- Cigarette smoke.
- Processed foods.
- Water that has coursed through galvanised mains.
- Industrial waste.
- Shellfish from polluted waters.
- Burning fossilised fuels.

Zinc seems to be important in counteracting some of the adverse effects of cadmium exposure.

Lead

Lead is associated with an increased risk of infertility, miscarriage, stillbirth, congenital abnormalities, fits, delayed development, reduced intelligence and early death. It tends to accumulate in the placenta and is present in higher amounts in babies born with deformity or stillbirth. We are exposed to lead from a number of sources:

- Exhaust fumes from lead in petrol.
- Water that has coursed through old lead water pipes, old lead-glazed earthenware mains or copper piping with alloy joins containing lead.
- Unlined tin cans.
- Food grown in polluted soil.
- Smoking tobacco treated with lead-containing insecticides.

Mercury

Exposure to excess mercury during pregnancy can cause miscarriage, cerebral palsy, mental retardation, blindness, fits, pre-term delivery and stillbirth.

Mercury crosses the placenta easily to be concentrated in the foetus – levels may be as much as 20 times higher in foetal compared with maternal blood. Our main sources of exposure to mercury are:

- Pesticides and fungicides.
- Fish (especially tuna) from polluted waters.
- Industrial waste.
- Dental amalgams.

All women who are following a pre-conceptual care programme, or who are pregnant, should avoid having dental treatment which involves the use of mercury-containing fillings. White fillings should be used instead.

The use of water filters

Water filters are now easily available and frequently used following saturation with network marketing schemes. Water filters undoubtedly improve the quality and taste of drinking water supplies. During your pre-conceptual care programme, it's worth considering the purchase of a water filter or using bottled mineral water instead. If you are not sure whether this is necessary, you can request that your local water board test your drinking water supplies for you.

If you are using a filter, ensure that the filter unit is changed at the frequency suggested by the manufacturer.

Hair mineral analysis

Hair mineral analysis is used as a method of detecting potentially harmful toxic metals in the body. Although by no means essential during the pre-conceptual care programme, it may help identify a problem if you find it difficult to conceive or if you suffer from recurrent miscarriages.

Farm chemicals

A study carried out in seven countries looked at the link between exposure to farm or agricultural chemicals and childhood cancers. When exposures were assessed in 1,218 children with a brain tumour and compared with 2,223 healthy children, it was found that those living on a farm with pigs, horses and/or cats were over three times more likely to develop a brain tumour than those not exposed. Maternal exposure during pregnancy and up to five years previously was associated with the greatest risk, especially if the mothers were employed as general farm workers. Agricultural chemicals, fertilisers, pesticides, animal manure and unprocessed wool were among the chemicals identified as potentially harmful.

Organophosphorus sheep dips

Organophosphorus sheep dips are dangerous to general human health as well as to the foetus. Even mild poisoning causes exhaustion, weakness, abdominal cramps, diarrhoea, excessive sweating and salivation in adults, plus constricted pupils for up to 24 hours after exposure.

Avoid any sheep dipping activity or contact with dipped sheep during your pre-conceptual care programme. At other times, always follow safety instructions (men as well as women), wear full protective clothing and obtain a certificate of competence for work with veterinary medicines.

Industrial chemicals

Toxins that are mainly responsible for environmental damage to the foetus's developing neurological system are by-products of the chlorine, plastics, electrical insulating and ink industries.

Polychlorinated biphenyls (PCBs) are now banned in Britain but are hard to eliminate as they were so widely used in industry. They are also resistant to biodegradation, one reason for their initial popularity. Burning plastic waste merely releases toxins such as dioxins and furans into the atmosphere, whilst dumping at sea would cause toxin accumulation in fatty fish. Dioxins from the atmosphere fall on to pasture land and rivers, thereby entering the food chain. Because they are fat soluble, they become concentrated in animal fat products such as meat, fish, milk, cheese, butter and cream.

Studies in the US looked at babies born to 313 mothers who had eaten dioxin-contaminated fish from Lake Michigan. The mothers had eaten an average of two or three trout or salmon from the lake each month over the sixteen years before their babies were born. Babies exposed to the highest concentrations of dioxin before birth were found to have lower birth weights and smaller head circumferences. They were also born six to twelve days earlier than those not exposed.

When examined for neurological deficits, almost half the exposed babies were relatively unresponsive, a third had jerky, uncoordinated movements and showed a greater tendency to suddenly startle. Four years later, these children were found to have impaired short-term memory.

Further studies involving 930 babies in North Carolina, USA, showed similar results. Extrapolation of data suggests that between 1 per cent and 8 per cent of British babies may be similarly affected as the body fat of British women shows similar levels of dioxins to that of US women.

Dioxins are also linked with miscarriages, congenital malformations, childhood and adult cancers, infant mortality and male infertility. The foetus is especially at risk of dioxins because:

- It lacks detoxification processes present after birth.
- Its small size means its intake of contaminants is disproportionately large.
- Cell division is occurring at a rapid rate during foetal development.

For information on the effects of dioxins on human sperm, see page 205.

It is important that everyone, especially those participating in a pre-conceptual care programme, should decrease their intake of dioxins. This is simply done by cutting down on consumption of animal fats, something that is already occurring during an active, pre-conceptual healthy eating plan. Skimmed or semi-skimmed milk is better than whole milk in this respect.

Other advice is to avoid obtaining all your dairy and meat products from one source and to avoid burning waste rubbish, especially plastics, during your pre-conceptual care programme and pregnancy. Even burning printing inks (e.g. on newspapers and magazines) can release dangerous toxins. Interestingly, one study has suggested that breast feeding appears to counteract the neurological effects of foetal dioxin contamination during pregnancy.

Tips to help detoxify your body

- Hair mineral analysis may indicate whether you have a particular toxic metal problem.
- Ensure an adequate intake of antioxidant vitamins and minerals – especially vitamins C, E and betacarotene, zinc, selenium, chromium and manganese. Vitamin C can lower body cadmium levels. Vitamins C and E, zinc and calcium can help reduce lead.
- Eat organic whole foods where possible.
- Avoid tinned foods, processed foods and excess salt.
- Eliminate all dietary additives.
- Wash all vegetables, fruit and salad stuff thoroughly.
- Garlic, yoghurt, bananas and pectin-containing fruit help to reduce absorption of dietary toxins.

- Avoid using aluminium kitchenware and foil. The effects of aluminium on long-term health are not yet known.
- Eliminate all non-essential drugs.
- Stop smoking and drinking alcohol.
- Reduce your intake of caffeine-containing drinks.
- Only have white dental fillings fitted.
- Consider either:
  – having your water supply analysed for toxic metals;
  – using a water filter; or
  – using bottled mineral water.
- Avoid heavy traffic and inhaling exhaust fumes. Keep car windows closed in traffic jams.
- Switch to using lead-free petrol and a car fitted with a catalytic converter.

Occupational risks

Some occupations involve exposure to chemical hazards, organophosphorus pesticides, solvents, formaldehyde, and industrial detergents/cleansers.

Abnormal sperm with large or small heads, or even two heads or tails, are found in higher than normal numbers in men who work in the lead, pesticide or chemical industries. These effects are similar to those seen in smokers and are thought to represent damage from oxidising free radical reactions (see page 101).

By ensuring a high intake of vitamins C, E and betacarotene – the antioxidant vitamins – some protection against environmental toxins may be provided (see page 101).

Workers in fossil fuel processing plants have increased risks of congenital abnormalities in their offspring.

Some research has suggested that women working in dry cleaners have a slightly increased risk of miscarriage. The risk is greatest for machine operators, who are more likely to miscarry than colleagues working in other parts of the business. The risk of a miscarriage in the general population is around 11 per cent. It rises to 15 per cent for women working in the dry cleaners but who don't operate machines, and to 18 per cent for women working as machine operators. The increased risk is thought to be caused by exposure to the solvent used as a dry cleaning agent. Exposure is apparently greatest when loading and unloading the machines and when cleaning button traps. If you are planning a baby, or are pregnant, tell your supervisor so your exposure to fumes can be reduced as much as possible.

X-rays

Most of us are now exposed to more irradiation than ever before through such things as airport security devices and medical investigations.

Exposure to ionising radiation, including X-rays, is a potent cause of genetic mutations in sperm and egg and of congenital malformations in the developing foetus.

Personnel exposed to radiation at work are protected by strict codes of conduct and wear radiation monitors.

Women at risk of exposure to radiation who wish to become pregnant should always seek the advice of their workplace medical officer early on during their pre-conceptual programme. Try to avoid having a routine X-ray during the pre-conceptual care period – and certainly if there is any chance that you are already pregnant.

VDUs – *visual display units*

Some studies have shown a link between using a VDU and an increased risk of miscarriage or foetal deformity. Statistical analysis suggests these links are anomalous rather than indicating a definite cause and effect.

A large study of 52,000 hospital deliveries in Canada in 1986 found the rate of malformations in the offspring of VDU users was 3.3 per cent compared with 3.7 per cent in non-users – i.e. the rate was actually reduced.

At present, the best advice is that using a VDU during pregnancy does not significantly increase the risk of foetal health problems. Women who work at a VDU screen are advised to ask their employers for ergonomically designed equipment such as chairs, wrist rests, feet rests and angled paper holders to reduce their risk of postural problems. Take frequent screen breaks, getting up to walk around your desk and stretch your arms and legs.

A consultation with an ergonomist will ensure that your typing posture is correct and that your desk, keyboard and screen are positioned at the optimum height for you.

15

Pre-conceptual genetic counselling

The location of our genes has now been fully mapped in the human genome project. This paves the way for increasingly accurate pre-conceptual genetic counselling. Pre-conception screening and counselling are available for many diseases that can run in families, such as sickle cell anaemia, thalassaemia, Tay Sachs disease, and cystic fibrosis. One in 20 of the population are carriers for the cystic fibrosis gene, for example, but are unaffected as they also possess a normal gene to balance it. If a child inherits two cystic fibrosis genes, however (a one in 400 risk), they develop the serious, life-limiting disease. Prenatal screening for cystic fibrosis appears to be most effective when 'couple screening' is used. This is because the result is only declared positive if both potential parents are found to be carriers. The couple can then be offered pre-implantation screening of embryos, or amniocentesis/chorionic villus sampling during early pregnancy (see pages 254 and 255). This reduces the number of false positives that occur when only the future mother is screened for. If her partner is not a carrier, the offspring will not be affected by cystic fibrosis.

Cousin marriage

Because cousins have each inherited some identical genes, the offspring of cousin marriages are more likely to inherit two abnormal genes (e.g. cystic fibrosis gene) and develop congenital abnormalities or diseases.

The risk of severe disability in the offspring of first cousins is one in 10 – three times higher than in the general population. This includes an increased risk of death before the age of five years.

Conversely, the chance of offspring being perfectly healthy is an acceptable 90 per cent – but couples who are blood relatives should strongly consider genetic counselling during their pre-conceptual care period.

Genetic counselling is also vital for any couple for whom there is a family history of an inherited (familial) disorder.

PART II
For future dads

16

Sperm and male reproductive health

It's vitally important that a potential father takes part in pre-conceptual care. Sperm are delicate cells. They are easily damaged and need careful nurturing to survive in sufficient numbers for fertilisation.

It takes an average of 74 days for the production of a mature sperm from its primitive germ cell. Sperm then take 20 days to traverse the 4- to 6-metre length of the tortuous epididymis during which they gain their motility. After this, they hang around in the vas deferens (the tube that's cut during vasectomy) for at least another six days before ejaculation. That's 100 days in which each sperm can undergo irreparable damage.

Once you've made the decision to have a baby, it makes sense to look after your sperm and increase the chance of a successful outcome.

It helps to have an idea of how sperm are formed before we look at the relatively simple ways to nurture them.

The formation of spermatozoa

Spermatozoa are made in a complicated yet elegant process called spermatogenesis.

The male testes consist of thousands of long, convoluted loops called seminiferous tubules. These tubules are lined by primitive germ cells known as spermatogonia which are equivalent to the primitive oogonia from which the female's eggs are made.

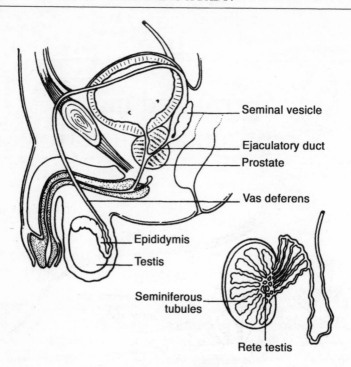

The male genito-urinary system

At adolescence, spermatogonia mature and start dividing to form primary spermatocytes. These cells enter a specialised form of division (meiosis) in which half the usual number of chromosomes go to each offspring cell (see diagram on page 9).

Meiosis is a two-stage process. During the first stage, the chromosomes double up and then pair off. The chromosomes exchange random blocks of genes within each pair. After exchanging genetic material, the paired chromosomes separate and the sperma-tocytes divide again. Each new cell now contains a different mix of genes, arranged in a different order on the 46 chromosomes, than are formed in any other body cells.

The second stage of meiosis now starts. The spermatocytes divide again, but this time each new cell only takes half the usual number of chromosomes. As a result, each new cell only contains 23

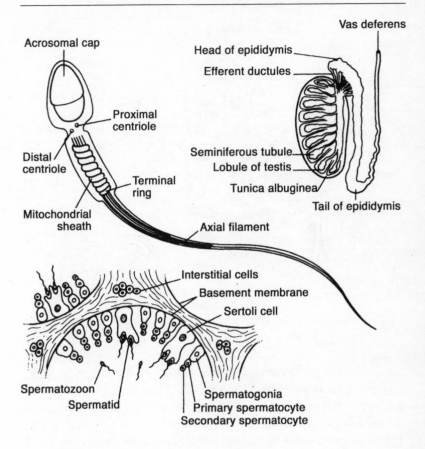

Spermatogenesis

chromosomes. All other male body cells contain 46 chromosomes.

Through this meiotic division, each original primary spermatocyte has now divided into four cells called spermatids. Each spermatid contains only half the genetic material found in the original primary spermatocyte. More importantly, each spermatid contains a unique set of genes – a random half selection from the parent cell. Some spermatids may have a similar selection of genes to other cells (accounting for family similarities between future brothers and sisters) but no two will ever be identical.

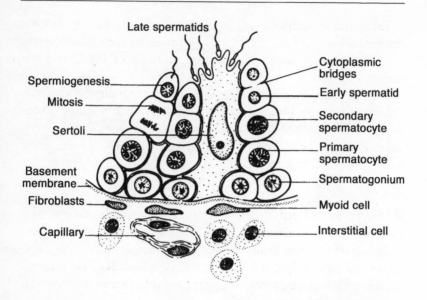

Spermatogonia, spermatocytes, spermatids and Sertoli cells

Each primitive germ cell (spermatogonium) continues to divide and may produce as many as 512 descendant spermatids. The process is so rapid that each testicle can produce an impressive 1,500 young sperm cells every second!

As the spermatids continue to mature and grow a tail, their heads become embedded in neighbouring nursery units – large, pyramidal cells called Sertoli cells. Here, they receive all the nutrients and hormones they need to develop into spermatozoa.

Once their tails are sufficiently developed, spermatozoa are released into the lumen of the seminiferous tubules but they are not yet fully mobile. They are propelled along by eddy currents in the surrounding seminiferous fluid – and also by the muscular contractions of ejaculation.

Sperm pass down the convoluted loops of the tubules, both ends of which drain into a network of ducts at the top of the testis. This network is called the epididymis and it is here that sperm finish growing their tail and start to acquire motility.

From the epididymis, sperm pass up into the top of the vas deferens where they are stored whilst completing their development – a process which we've already seen takes up to 100 days from start to finish.

During orgasm, sperm are pumped up through the two vas deferens, over the bladder and into the ejaculatory ducts. These ducts actually pass through the prostate gland so that sperm spill out into the urethra, along with secretions from the seminal vesicles within the prostate gland itself.

Sertoli cells

The large Sertoli cells line the seminiferous tubules where they alternate with the primitive germ cells from which sperm develop.

Developing sperm heads become embedded in these large cells, rather like tiny tadpoles in aspic jelly. The Sertoli cells secrete a number of hormones, proteins, sugars and other nutrients that help their lodgers to mature.

Sertoli cells have an important extra function. They interlock tightly on the inner membrane of the seminiferous tubules to form what is known as the blood-testis barrier. Rather like a rubber ground sheet, this barrier prevents large molecules seeping from surrounding blood capillaries into the central space of the seminiferous tubules.

The blood-testis barrier is vital. It allows the nutrient fluid inside the seminiferous tubules to maintain its high concentration of sex hormones, potassium salts and certain acids. It also protects young sperm from attack by blood-borne infections or poisonous molecules.

Perhaps the most important function of the blood-testis barrier is that it prevents sperm fragments (formed during development) from accidentally entering the circulation and triggering the formation of anti-sperm antibodies.

If the barrier is disrupted for any reason so that sperm and blood are mixed (e.g. by external injury to the testicle; during vasectomy) a man may start to make antibodies against his own sperm, resulting in subfertility.

Interestingly, when the primitive germ cells divide, the resultant cells must pass through the blood-testis barrier as they mature and travel towards the tubular lumen. This seems to occur without disrupting the barrier. Adjacent Sertoli cells form new tight junctions below the moving germ cells while, at the same time, releasing the connections above.

Testosterone and its importance

At puberty, the testes are switched on by two hormones secreted in the pituitary gland at the base of the brain. These two hormones are follicle stimulating hormone (FSH) and luteinising hormone (LH).

FSH triggers the production and development of sperm by stimulating the Sertoli cells. LH promotes the production of the male hormone testosterone. Testosterone is responsible for the male secondary sex characteristics that occur at puberty and is essential for sperm production.

In each testis, the spaces between the convoluted seminiferous tubules are filled with little nests of cells – the interstitial cells of Leydig. These contain fatty granules rich in cholesterol from which testosterone is made.

The effects of testosterone on reproduction

* Male sex drive.
* Growth of the penis, testes and scrotum.
* Growth of the seminal vesicles and secretion of fluids rich in the sugar fructose.
* Growth of the prostate gland and secretion of prostatic fluids making up a third of semen volume.
* Maturation of spermatids to spermatozoa while embedded in Sertoli cells.

The prostate gland

The healthy prostate gland is the size and shape of a large chestnut. It weighs up to 20 g and is situated beneath the bladder, wrapped around the urethra.

Why the prostate exists at all is not fully understood. It is made up of muscle and fibre cells plus millions of tiny glands. These glands release their secretions into the urethra during ejaculation, providing up to 30 per cent of semen by volume. It is the prostatic secretions (and its proteins: spermine, spermidine and putrescine) which give semen its characteristic smell.

Although prostatic secretions are thought to keep sperm healthy, they are not essential for reproduction. Sperm which have not come into contact with prostate fluid can still fertilise an egg.

What does prostate fluid contain?

- Water.
- Salts.
- Minerals (calcium, phosphorus, magnesium, zinc, copper).
- Proteins.
- Antibodies.
- Enzymes.
- Citric acid.
- Lipids (fats).
- Prostaglandins (hormone-like chemicals).

Another possible role for the prostate gland is to direct semen outwards during ejaculation so sperm don't reflux up into the bladder.

Erection

Erections are involuntary, nervous reflexes controlled by the spinal cord. They are usually triggered by physical stimulation of the penis or by erotic thoughts. Most men experience between one and five erections while asleep. These last around half an hour each and are often in evidence on waking.

The human penis contains no muscle or bone. It maintains a rigid erection by trapping blood under tension in three expandable cylinders of tissue: two corpora cavernosa and one corpus spongiosum. An erection is initiated by dilation of small arteries in the penis. Blood rushes into the penis and is shunted into the three cylinders of tissue, which rapidly engorge. They expand in the same way as empty balloons filling with water.

As the cylinders expand, they press on veins taking blood away from the penis, blocking outflow. Blood is now trapped in the penis and, as more blood flows in, the pressure goes up. This produces a rigid erection and also helps prevent urination during engorgement. In effect, the penis has its own hydrostatic skeleton – a mechanism also relied on by lower life forms such as the garden earthworm.

Ejaculation

Ejaculation is another nervous reflex controlled by the spinal cord. It occurs in two parts:

- Emission, in which semen moves through the ejaculatory ducts (running through the prostate gland) and into the central tube of the penis – the urethra.
- Ejaculation proper, in which semen is propelled out of the urethra by contraction of pelvic muscles.

Semen

Semen is a white-yellow, opalescent secretion which is thick and clotted. It consists mainly of fluids from the testis and epididymis, seminal vesicles and prostate gland with some contributions from other small glands such as Cowper's gland. Sperm form only a small fraction of semen by volume – less than 20 per cent. The average volume of semen ejaculated after a few days of abstinence is 3.5 ml, though this can rise to 13 ml if sexual activity has not occurred for several weeks.

More than 32 different chemicals are found in semen, including fructose sugar, vitamin C, vitamin E, vitamin B12, sulphur, zinc and potassium. Hormone-like chemicals, prostaglandins, are secreted into the semen by the prostate gland and seminal vesicles. They have a number of actions, including causing the female's womb to contract. In obstetrics, prostaglandin pessaries are used to ripen the cervix of a pregnant woman, which induces labour.

Prostaglandins in semen are thought to make the female cervix open and pout so sperm can swim through more easily. It's possible they also make the female orgasm more intense and help sperm travel up the female reproductive tract in eddy currents.

Spermatozoa

Spermatozoa (singular: spermatozoon) are fascinating things. Even though it only takes one sperm to fertilise an egg, semen normally contains 100 million sperm per millilitre – an average of 330 million sperm per ejaculation. This figure can rise to over 1,000 million spermatozoa in any one ejaculate. Each sperm measures 0.05 mm in length and has a so-called head, middle piece and tail.

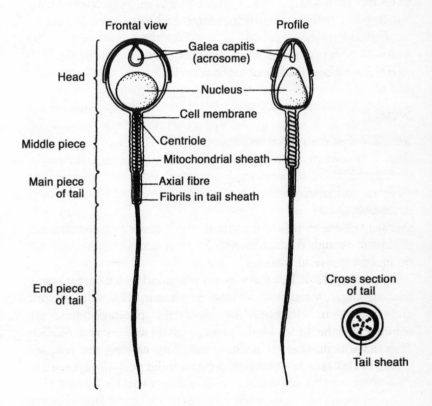

Human sperm

The sperm head is shaped like a flattened tear-drop. The front snout contains a sac of enzymes, the acrosome. These enzymes are essential for fertilisation and help the sperm dissolve the coating of an egg to allow penetration. Behind the acrosome is the cell nucleus, containing a random half set of a man's genetic material (DNA) tightly coiled in 23 chromosomes.

Each sperm possesses a unique set of genetic information, which, although it may be similar to the genetic information in another sperm from the same male, will never be exactly the same.

The middle piece is really the fattest part of the sperm tail. Its extra thickness is a result of small power units – the mitochondria – which are wrapped around the tail in a spiral sheath. Mitochondria produce the energy for sperm motility by burning fructose sugar which is found in semen in large quantities.

The tail is made up of 20 long filaments – a central pair surrounded by two rings each containing nine fibrils. At the front end of the tail is a further ring of thicker fibres and also a protective tail sheath. This sheath peters out further down the sperm until only a thin cell membrane encloses the end of the tail. This gradual thinning and tapering of the tail helps the sperm produce its whiplash-like swimming motion.

Facts about sperm

- Sperm are produced at a rate of 1,500 per second from each testicle.
- Sperm take 74 days to form and a further 26 days to mature.
- Sperm swim at a rate of 3 mm per hour.
- A sperm lashes its tail 800 times to swim one centimetre.
- Sperm reach the Fallopian tubes within 30 to 60 minutes after ejaculation into the female tract, helped along by eddy currents.
- Sperm can normally only survive in the vagina for up to six hours due to the acidity of vaginal secretions.
- The average survival time for a sperm in the female reproductive tract is three to four days.
- On rare occasions, viable sperm have survived for as long as a week in the female reproductive tract. Whether or not they are capable of fertilisation is unknown.

Capacitation

By the time sperm are ejaculated, most are fully motile. Interestingly, the longer time they spend in the female genital tract, the greater their ability to fertilise an egg.

The sperm become stickier and better able to adhere to the outside of the egg. This process is known as capacitation and is probably triggered by female secretions. Sperm can also be capacitated by incubation with tissue fluids – a technique which increases the chance of successful artificial insemination.

Sperm counts and fertility

As a general rule, 50 per cent of men with sperm counts of 20 to 40 million per ml are subfertile and men with a sperm count lower than 20 million per ml are essentially sterile. So, even if a man produces a teaspoon (5 ml) of semen containing 100 million sperm, his chances of fathering a child are slim.

This is not an absolute rule, however, and doctors should always be wary of telling any infertile couple with a poor semen analysis that the husband is infertile. One man with a sperm count as low as 50,000 per ml, of which only 10 per cent were motile, has fathered a child. Genetic analysis proves he is 99.99 per cent certain to be the biological father.

Another study suggests that a low sperm count just increases the average number of monthly cycles it takes for the female partner to conceive:

Motile sperm count (millions/ml)	Average number cycles to conceive
<5	11
5–20	9.4
20–60	8
>60	6

Studies with couples investigated for subfertility show that the eventual chance of conception is related to the number of sperm that are motile. When there are fewer than five to ten million motile sperm per ml the chance of eventually conceiving is 30 per cent. When the motile sperm count is greater than 100 million per ml, the chance of success rises to 70 per cent.

So in general, the higher the sperm count and the higher the percentage of motile sperm, the higher the chance of conception – but even men with counts in the presumed sterile range are capable of naturally fathering a child.

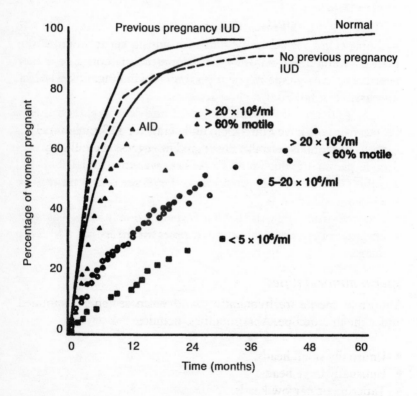

Graph of percentage chance of pregnancy in relation to sperm count over 5 years (IUD = intra-uterine device, AID = artificial insemination by donor)

Sperm have a difficult task. The distance and conditions under which they have to travel are comparable to a person swimming the English Channel – assuming it were filled with treacle.

Even when a man ejaculates 300 million sperm near the female cervix, only 50 to 150 sperm eventually reach the upper Fallopian tube. This is where fertilisation of the descending egg occurs.

The other 299,999,850 sperm become lost on the way. One theory is these excess sperm are needed to overwhelm the female's immune system so it doesn't attack the successfully invading sperm.

To quote Monty Python's *The Meaning of Life*, every sperm is sacred.

Falling sperm counts

It is vital that a man does everything in his power to improve the quality and quantity of his sperm during the pre-conceptual care period. The average sperm count is rapidly dwindling. Over the last 50 years:

- Sperm counts have fallen from an average of 113 million per ml to 66 million per ml. Recent studies suggest the fall may have been less dramatic, to 76 million per ml.
- Semen volume has dropped from an average of 3.4 ml to 2.75 ml.
- Sperm motility has decreased.
- The percentage of sperm with abnormal structure has increased.

Sperm abnormalities

Abnormal sperm are frequently found when semen is examined under the microscope. Abnormalities include:

- Unusually small heads.
- Unusually large heads.
- Tapering or narrow heads.
- Two heads and one tail.
- One head and two tails.
- Sluggishness.

- Tendency to swim in circles.
- Erratic zig-zag swimming pattern.
- Sperm clumping together (agglutination).

It is estimated that as many as 10 per cent of sperm can be abnormal without loss of fertility. It is now considered normal, however, to find up to 40 per cent of sperm in the ejaculate with structural abnormalities.

Between 1977 and 1989 the number of men with low sperm counts tripled, while those with reduced sperm motility doubled from 21 per cent to 43 per cent. At the same time, researchers have noted a twelve-fold increase in the numbers of abnormal sperm. Why is this, and what can men do to protect themselves from an ever-falling sperm count?

The following pages examine all the factors that can affect sperm count adversely. By knowing what these are, men can take positive steps to improve the quality and quantity of their sperm during their pre-conceptual care programme.

17

Factors that significantly affect sperm formation

Effect of temperature on sperm formation

The testicles seem unusually vulnerable. They start their development near the kidneys but go out of their way to descend through the abdomen and drop into the scrotal bag. Other important parts of the anatomy – e.g. the brain and heart – have evolved within protective bony cages. Strangely, the testicles are offered no protection against rugby scrums or ungentlemanly tackles. Why?

The answer has to do with temperature. Spermatogenesis, the 100-day sperm production line, requires a lower temperature than normal body heat. By hanging the washing out of the window, so to speak, the testes are kept at a cool 32°C – a significant 5°C below core body temperature of 37°C.

The testes achieve this temperature drop through air circulating round the scrotum – and probably by a sophisticated mechanism exchanging heat between the spermatic arteries which take blood away.

If the testicles are warmed for continuous periods of time (e.g. by failing to descend from the abdomen, or by tight, hot underwear) sperm counts fall significantly.

In humans, it has been found experimentally that taking a hot bath (43°C to 45°C) for only half an hour a day can also lower sperm counts – as can wearing tight athletic scrotal supports.

Another study looked at the effects of wearing loose or tight underwear on the semen quality of two adult males. Although only

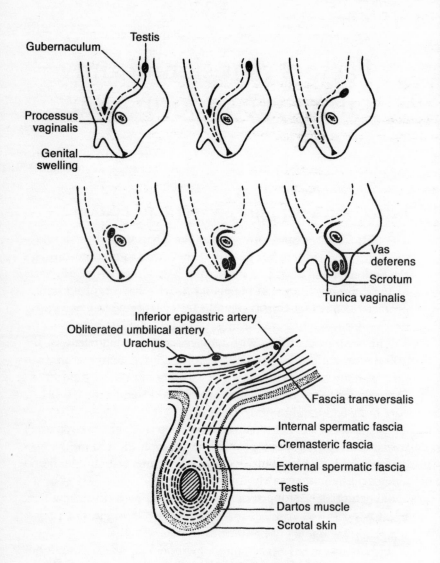

Descent of testes through inguinal canal

a small study, it is further scientific evidence (as opposed to popular folklore) that the fit of a man's underwear can affect his sperm. Both men were participants in a sperm bank programme, so their normal semen analyses were well documented.

Both men wore tight, bikini-type briefs for three months and then changed to loose boxer shorts for three months. They then repeated this tight-loose sequence once more.

Results were quite impressive. Total sperm count and density plus sperm motility gradually decreased while the men wore tight briefs and gradually increased when wearing loose boxer shorts. Changes appeared to start within two weeks of changing over to each new set of underwear, which was much faster than was expected.

The first male provided an average of one semen sample per week. The second male delivered approximately two specimens per week. The men each started the programme at different times to exclude any seasonal variations. The results were as follows:

	First male			Second male		
Variable	Tight	Loose	Percentage change	Tight	Loose	Percentage change
Total sperm/ ejaculation (millions)	242	301	+20%	411	465	+13%
Sperm density (millions/ml)	77	86	+10%	148	177	+16%
Total motile (millions)	193	239	+21%	291	343	+15%
Volume (ml)	3.1	3.5	+12%	2.5	2.7	+7%

Source: Sanger and Friman, *Reproductive Toxicology*, 1990, Vol 4, pp 229–232.

The clear conclusion is that during the pre-conceptual care period at least, men should wear loose-fitting boxer shorts rather than tight, bikini-style briefs.

Effect of electrostatic electricity

Tight polyester underwear generates electrostatic electricity caused by friction between the synthetic material and scrotal skin.

Recent studies show that polyester underpants generate enough electrostatic charges to create an electrostatic field. This can cross the scrotal wall to have a potentially devastating effect on male fertility. Thirty-three males were studied for 18 months:

- In the group wearing polyester underwear, four out of eleven men showed evidence of a significant reduction in sperm count plus testicular *degeneration* – i.e. serious damage – by the fourteenth month. This change was reversed when the underpants were discarded.
- In the group wearing polyester-cotton mix underwear, only one out of eleven showed a low sperm count by the sixteenth month. This change was reversed when the underpants were discarded.
- In the group wearing pure cotton underpants, no significant changes in sperm were noted.

In all cases, no significant changes were found in testicular temperature or blood hormone levels. Changes were attributed to the electrostatic field generated.

Another study compared the electrostatic potentials generated in three groups of healthy volunteers who wore underpants made from cotton, polyester or a 50 per cent polyester 50 per cent cotton mix. No electrostatic potentials were detected when cotton pants were worn. The pure polyester pants generated the highest potentials whilst the polyester-cotton pants generated readings half as high.

Another clear conclusion is that in the pre-conceptual care period at least, men should wear cotton pants.

Effect of temperature and electrostatic forces combined

A polyester jockstrap was devised as a method of male contraception. A scrotal sling was tailored to enclose the testicles while allowing the penis to poke through. A belt attached to the sling fitted round the waist and pulled the testicles up close to the abdomen. The sling was worn day and night and only changed when soiled.

Egyptian doctors found the sperm counts of all 14 volunteers dropped to *zero* and remained at zero after an average of 140 days wearing the sling. The volume of semen produced also fell significantly. These effects were the result of a combination of electrostatic charges and increased local heat. The higher the temperature, the greater the electrostatic field.

Once a male produced three semen samples in which no sperm were found, his female partner stopped using her hormonal method of contraception. None of the women conceived during the remainder of the 12-month study.

Once the slings were discarded, the men's sperm counts climbed back up to previous normal levels within an average of 157 days. All five couples who then planned to conceive after the study did so – with four normal live births resulting plus, sadly, one spontaneous miscarriage.

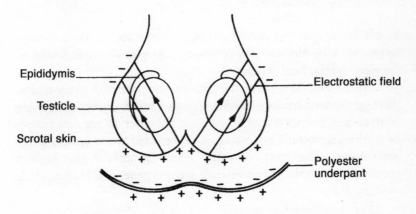

Electrostatic charge across sling/scrotum

Seasonal effects

The quality of semen is lower in summer than in winter. In one study, regular sperm counts were performed on 131 volunteers. Although the volume of semen produced by each male did not vary significantly, the total sperm count per ejaculation fell from 320 million in winter to 250 million at the height of summer – July and August. This effect may have a number of causes:

- Seasonal dietary differences.
- Temperature variations.
- Environmental pollution levels.
- Atmospheric radiation levels.
- Hormonal variations.
- Activity and lifestyle differences between summer and winter e.g. sport; use of saunas.
- Varying stress levels.

Given that it takes around 100 days to produce a sperm from start to finish, any event that lowers sperm counts in July might have a basis in something occurring in April to May. Traditionally, men's thoughts are supposed to turn to love in spring. Perhaps this is evidence to the contrary.

Stress

It has been known for years that stress affects sperm production. During the Second World War, Nazi doctors subjected Jewish prisoners to barbaric stress by successively firing blank cartridges at them. The prisoners rapidly stopped making sperm and counts fell to zero.

Men today are subjected to increasing levels of stress throughout their daily lives:

- Pressure to succeed.
- Long, tiring days at work.
- Endlessly ringing phones.

- Office noise levels.
- Traffic jams.
- Financial worries.
- Increasing risk of violence.

The list is endless. Some experts believe that the falling sperm count is nature's way of dealing with the pressures of twentieth-century life and urban population overgrowth. During the pre-conceptual programme it is important that both partners find time to relax.

Toxins and pollutants

One expert who specialises in the effects of industrialisation has suggested that society is conducting a big experiment, exposing whole cities to high levels of pollution – especially in Eastern Europe. As a result, it is possible that the falling sperm count has environmental origins. These include:

- Workplace exposure to chemicals and toxins.
- Toxic substances from industry.
- Thinning ozone layer and increasing radiation.
- Nonionic detergents in sewage effluent. These are already thought to affect male fish so they behave like females – producing a primitive yolk (vitellogenin).
- Polychlorinated biphenyls (PCBs) – a group of weakly oestrogenic chemicals banned since 1970. Prior to this, they were widely used as electrical insulators. Because of their high toxicity, they have persisted in the atmosphere and accumulated in the food chain, especially in animal fats. Certainly studies of animals suggest that PCBs can impair male fertility, though this has not yet been proven in men (see page 175).
- Oestrogens in the environment.

Effects of environmental oestrogens on male fertility

Oestrogen is a natural female hormone essential for female fertility, pregnancy and the development of female characteristics.

Between 1945 and 1971, several million pregnant women were prescribed high doses of the synthetic oestrogen diethylstilboestrol (DES), to prevent a threatened miscarriage. The sons of those women were born with a greater risk of birth defects, including undescended testicles, an abnormal penis and the future development of testicular cancer.

At maturity, these males also produced lower than normal semen volumes and low sperm counts. The effects were all thought to be caused by exposure to the artificial female hormone, DES, while in the womb.

Over the last 30 to 50 years, these same birth defects have become more common in men who have not knowingly been exposed to synthetic oestrogens in the womb. At the same time, semen volume and sperm counts have fallen dramatically. It is suggested that weak, synthetic oestrogens in the environment are at fault. Is this possible? The answer seems to be yes.

The increased use of synthetic chemicals and changes in our diet over the last 50 years have led some experts to claim we are now living in 'a virtual sea of oestrogen'. Modern environmental pollutants such as PCBs and detergents seem to mimic oestrogen and are thought to damage the male reproductive system while it is still developing in the mother's womb. Continuing exposure to oestrogens throughout early life affects sperm formation. One theory is that weak environmental oestrogens inhibit the division of testicular Sertoli cells before puberty. If you remember, Sertoli cells are the nursery cells in which sperm become embedded while maturing (see page 189). Each Sertoli cell can only support a certain number of sperm. So fewer Sertoli cells mean a lower sperm count.

Another theory is that exposure to oestrogen inhibits the development of testicular Leydig cells. These cells secrete testosterone which is responsible for masculinising the developing male reproductive tract. Fewer Leydig cells mean less testosterone during development and an increased risk of abnormal development, e.g. undescended testicles, lower sperm count at maturity. These effects can be shown experimentally in animals such as rats.

Men are exposed to oestrogens through:

- Foods – plant and fungal hormones (phytoestrogens), e.g. soya, rye extract, fungi.
  - use of anabolic oestrogens in livestock. This was banned in Europe in 1981, but was an important source of exposure in the 1950s to 1970s.
  - increased intake of dairy products: cows' milk contains natural oestrogens as cows continue to lactate while pregnant.
- Body fat – which can convert other steroid hormones into oestrogen. In Britain, 45 per cent of males are now overweight and 8 per cent are obese.
- Pollutants such as PCBs, dioxins, dichloro-diphenyl trichloroethane (DDT). The exhaust gases from petrol engines also contain oestrogen-like chemicals.
- Traces of drugs (e.g. contraceptive Pills; HRT) in drinking water.

Environmental oestrogens are already affecting wildlife. Researchers in Florida, for example, have found a significant change in the male:female sex ratio of reptiles inhabiting polluted lakes.

It is certain that both pregnant women and mature men are exposed to more oestrogens now than we were 50 years ago. This could well explain decreasing male fertility. It is thought that this environmental exposure, even though it is weak, has a more potent effect on the male foetus than on the adult male.

Diet and sperm

Our diet is important. To quote an old chestnut, 'We are what we eat.'

We are also a summation of all the metabolic changes that occur in our bodies every day. Unfortunately, many of these reactions are harmful – to sperm and eggs as well as other cells. Our diet plays a large part in protecting us from ourselves by supplying antioxidant vitamins and minerals to neutralise harmful reactions.

The effects of free radicals

It is estimated that 40 per cent of sperm damage is caused by the harmful effects of free radicals.

A free radical is an unstable molecule which has a negative

charge. It seeks to neutralise this charge by colliding with other molecules and stealing one or more positive charges. This process is called oxidation.

Oxidating collisions generate new free radicals from molecules that have lost their positive charge. In this way, a chain reaction is triggered. Electric charges are passed to and fro, with most free radicals only existing for microseconds at a time.

Free radicals are usually rapidly mopped up and neutralised (e.g. by reducing enzymes or antioxidants) but they still cause considerable damage to cell membranes, intercellular proteins and our genetic material, DNA. In fact, free radical damage is so severe that it is linked with many types of cancer, heart disease, cataracts and premature wrinkling of the skin.

It has been estimated that every cell in our body – including sperm and eggs – is attacked by 10,000 free radical oxidising reactions every day (see page 101 for further details).

Sperm and free radicals

Most men have 20 per cent to 40 per cent obviously abnormal sperm when semen is examined in the laboratory. Many more will have genetic abnormalities that remain undetected. As stated before, 40 per cent of these abnormalities are thought to result from collisions between free radicals and sperm.

Damage to DNA can result in the wrong nucleotide (one of the units making up the DNA strand) bases being inserted when the DNA sequence is read. If this occurs in a dividing germ cell destined to produce a sperm, a mutation results, which may cause subfertility, birth defects, genetic diseases or childhood cancers in resultant offspring from that sperm.

Sperm and genetic abnormalities

Genetic abnormalities in the offspring are more frequently associated with faults in paternal DNA (from the sperm) than defects in maternal genes (derived from the egg). This is probably because of the greater number of cell divisions (mitoses) needed to form a sperm – an estimated 380 compared with only 23 cell divisions needed to produce an egg.

Cell division is a time when genetic accidents – such as faulty DNA sequence insertion – are most likely to occur. Chromosomes are actively replicating and cellular repair mechanisms are inactivated during this phase.

A good example of a paternally linked cancer is that of the retina at the back of the eye (retinoblastoma). This tumour affects one out of every 20,000 babies born in the UK every year. All the cells in infants developing this serious disease lack a part of one chromosome (in chromosome pair number 13). This genetic defect is more commonly linked to an abnormality inherited from the sperm rather than a faulty egg.

Vitamin C and sperm health

Our main protection against free radicals generated by our metabolic reactions are antioxidant substances found in our diet. These include vitamin C, vitamin E, betacarotene, garlic, some minerals and even substances found in red wine.

Vitamin C is a water-soluble antioxidant. It is actively secreted into semen and is present at concentrations eight times higher than those found in the blood.

Vitamin C plays a dual role in protecting sperm. Semen contains a substance called non-specific sperm agglutinin. This is made up of a protein, a sugar, vitamin E, plus several sulphur-containing groups. This substance exists in either an oxidised or a non-oxidised (reduced) form. When in the reduced form, it binds to sperm heads (through its sulfhydryl groups) and prevents sperm clumping together. This increases sperm motility. When it exists in its oxidised form, it can't bind to sperm and sperm therefore stick to each other. This causes them to clump and become immobile. If 20 per cent or more of sperm are clumped together, infertility usually occurs. Vitamin C, by acting as an antioxidant, keeps the agglutinin in its reduced form so it can bind to sperm.

In one study, 35 infertile men were given 500 mg of vitamin C every twelve hours (i.e. twice a day) for one month. After only one week, the average percentage of sperm clumped together had dropped from 37 per cent to 14 per cent. After two weeks, sperm agglutination had dropped to 13 per cent and at four weeks was down to 11 per cent.

As this study proceeded, the researchers confirmed a significant improvement in overall quality of the men's sperm, including percentage of normal sperm present, sperm viability and sperm motility.

Later research also shows that vitamin C protects the genetic material (DNA) of sperm against the oxidising reactions of free radicals. This reduces the risk of siring offspring with an inherited genetic disease. Both of these actions (anti-clumping and anti-oxidant) are important in maintaining sperm quality and the power to fertilise an egg.

In one interesting trial, a chemical resulting from damaged DNA was measured in the sperm of men on a relatively high vitamin C diet – 250 mg per day. The vitamin C in their diet was then drastically reduced to only 5 mg per day. The level of the chemical resulting from DNA damage promptly doubled.

The researchers believe this proves that vitamin C protects against sperm damage. They then upped the vitamin C level in their male volunteers to 10 mg and then 20 mg per day – to no effect. Levels of vitamin C in the sperm of volunteers continued to fall. It wasn't until the daily intake of vitamin C rose to 250 mg per day that the protective effect returned.

Blood levels of vitamin C are high in followers of the Mediterranean diet, whereas levels in some inhabitants of the UK are low enough to put them at risk of scurvy.

Vitamin C is one of the most delicate nutrients in the diet. It is easily destroyed by oxygen, metal ions (e.g. from saucepans and utensils), increased pH (alkalinity), heat and even light.

Good dietary sources are fruits (citrus, guava, peppers, paw-paw, mangoes, berries, kiwi fruit) and sprouting vegetables such as broccoli.

The European reference nutrient intake of vitamin C is 60 mg per day. This is based on the amounts needed to protect against vitamin C deficiency disease (scurvy) and to maintain healthy tissues. Many experts now believe that we need much higher levels of vitamin C for its protective antioxidant effects. Vitamin C mops up free radicals and is also essential to regenerate antioxidant vitamin E.

Study after study shows that high blood levels of vitamin C protect against coronary heart disease and cancer and may even prolong life.

While preparing to father a child, I would strongly recommend that men maintain a high vitamin C intake of at least 250 mg per day. This means eating at least two portions of fruit and three servings of raw or lightly steamed vegetables per day.

Although diet should always come first as a vitamin source, taking a daily food supplement of 150 mg to 250 mg of vitamin C per day in tablet form can only do good. Vitamin C plays a vital first-defence role in protecting the genetic material in sperm – and therefore in protecting your future offspring.

Smokers need to obtain at least twice as much vitamin C as non-smokers. Their blood levels of vitamin C are up to 40 per cent lower than those of non-smokers and sperm abnormalities are greater (see page 217).

Vitamin E and sperm

Vitamin E is a powerful antioxidant vitamin. Unlike vitamin C it is fat soluble, which means it can penetrate cell membranes and body fats to protect them against oxidising free radical attacks.

Trials have proven that high blood levels of vitamin E are linked with a reduced risk of coronary heart disease. It is also thought that low blood levels increase the risk of developing cancer.

The reference nutrient intake for vitamin E is 10 mg per day. This is based on providing enough vitamin E to prevent oxidation of polyunsaturated fats in our diet. A diet rich in vitamin E will provide around 20 mg per day. Many experts now believe we need 40 mg to 50 mg per day to protect against free radical attack. Smokers may need as much as 60 mg per day.

Vitamin E is found naturally in vegetable oils, seeds, avocado, wheatgerm, nuts and seafood. The richest source is wheatgerm oil, providing 136 mg per 100 g.

Vitamin E is now being tested as a treatment for infertility in men. Superoxide free radicals are present in semen, where they are

produced by white blood cells and also from the process of spermatogenesis itself. High levels of superoxide radicals in semen are
linked with subfertility. Researchers believe a high dietary intake of
vitamin E will mop up these superoxide radicals and increase fertility.

Vitamin E is also needed for the flexibility of sperm cell walls,
which is important in motility. As we saw above, the agglutinin
molecule that coats sperm to prevent them clumping together also
contains vitamin E. Vitamin E plays an important role in preventing
sperm clumping and promoting motility. The agglutinin molecule,
and vitamin E itself, are maintained in a non-oxidised form by
vitamin C. It is therefore wise to take vitamin C supplements as well
as vitamin E during the pre-conceptual care period at least.

Betacarotene and sperm

Betacarotene is converted in the body to vitamin A (a powerful
antioxidant) when vitamin A stores are low. Otherwise, it remains
as betacarotene, a powerful antioxidant in its own right. As excess
vitamin A is poisonous, ensuring an adequate intake of betacarotene is the safest way to maintain optimal blood levels.

Betacarotene and other carotenoids are found in dark green
leaves such as spinach and broccoli, and also in yellow-orange
fruits or vegetables such as sweet potatoes, carrots, red/yellow
capsicums, apricots and mangoes.

As carotenoids are water soluble they are likely to protect sperm
in semen from free radical attack in a similar way to vitamin C.

Zinc and sperm

As an antioxidant, zinc is important in protecting sperm against free
radical attack (see page 101). Recent research shows it has other
effects that are important for optimum male fertility. Each ejaculate
contains around 5 mg of zinc – one third of the recommended
nutrient intake.

Seminal zinc is known to keep sperm in a quiescent state, with
energy conservation and reduced oxygen consumption. Within the
female tract, zinc levels are low and seminal zinc rapidly diffuses
away. This triggers the sperm to speed up and become almost
supercharged as they dash to find the egg.

Zinc also protects sperm DNA (chromatin) from breaking down and has a significant effect on the structure of human sperm protamines – proteins that condense 85 per cent of sperm DNA into an insoluble and stable complex. If sperm chromatin is not kept in this condensed form, successful fertilisation is unlikely.

When a sperm meets an egg, it releases enzymes from a sac at the sperm head which digest the outer egg coating and allow the sperm to penetrate. This is known as the 'acrosome reaction'. Sometimes these enzymes are discharged spontaneously and too early, which effectively renders a sperm incapable of fertilisation. High concentrations of zinc have been shown to damp down the acrosome reaction, probably by altering membrane permeability to potassium. This effect is reversible, so when zinc concentrations are reduced in the female tract, the acrosome reaction can again occur. This mechanism reduces the chance of a spontaneous acrosome reaction occurring before the sperm reaches the egg and fertilisation can take place. For all these reasons, it is important that a man has an adequate intake of zinc throughout the pre-conceptual care period (see page 99).

Selenium and sperm

The mineral selenium is needed for normal testosterone metabolism and testicular development in males. A unique selenium-containing protein found in sperm cells is essential for sperm motility, and subfertile men with low selenium levels can significantly improve their chances of conception by taking selenium supplements. In one study, 69 men were divided into three groups, one of which received selenium alone, one took selenium plus antioxidants and the other took an inactive placebo for three months. In both groups receiving selenium, sperm motility doubled from 17.5 per cent to 35.1 per cent, and 11 per cent of men receiving selenium successfully fathered a child compared with no change and no conceptions in the placebo group.

Antioxidant recommendations for pre-conceptual care

Bearing in mind that it takes 100 days to make a mature, motile sperm – and that it takes around 30 ejaculations to flush through pre-formed sperm already in the vas deferens – it seems reasonable to take antioxidant vitamin supplements (C, E, selenium and carotenoids) for at least three months prior to conceiving, and preferably six.

If you want to protect yourself against coronary heart disease and future cancers, many experts would recommend that you continue taking antioxidant supplements for the rest of your life.

Alcohol and sperm

As Shakespeare noted, alcohol 'provokes the desire but takes away the performance' (*Macbeth*, II:3).

As well as inducing brewer's droop, excess alcohol consumption reduces the production of spermatozoa. The breakdown product of alcohol metabolism, acetaldehyde, is also a cellular poison that is toxic to sperm.

As much as 40 per cent of male infertility is linked to alcohol intake, even just a moderate amount. The main effect of alcohol is to interfere with testosterone secretion so levels fall. It also hastens testosterone breakdown in the body, accelerating its conversion to oestrogen. As we've already seen, increased blood levels of oestrogen are associated with a significant lowering of sperm counts (see page 205). In addition, the lower than normal blood testosterone level results in a decreased sex drive.

It's now thought that up to 40 per cent of male subfertility is caused by moderate alcohol intake. The good news is that this effect is reversible. Out of 67 men attending a hospital infertility clinic, 26 (39 per cent) had a low sperm count. They had all been investigated by fertility specialists in the past and no cause for the infertility had been found.

When the men were advised to stop drinking alcohol, the sperm counts of half of them returned to normal within three months. The number of motile sperm increased significantly and the numbers of abnormal forms also dropped. As a result, at least ten men (78 per cent of those whose sperm counts responded) successfully fathered a child.

UK *units*

The healthy weekly alcohol limit for men is 21 units, with 50 units or more being dangerous. (For examples of alcohol units see page 162.)

Most drinkers tend to over-estimate the strength of spirits and under-estimate the strength of beer. For example, a man drinking two pints of beer has consumed *four* units. A man drinking two glasses of wine and a double vodka has also consumed *four* units.

Excessive alcohol weakens heart muscle. Men who drink more than three pints a day (six units) are at twice the risk of sudden cardiac death than those drinking moderately (two to four units). Binge drinkers and those who drink heavily only at weekends and holidays are also at increased risk.

Smoking and sperm

There is growing evidence that smoking cigarettes affects not only the health of the man himself, but also the future health of his offspring.

Fathers who smoke are more likely to produce offspring who die young (e.g. cot death) or are born with genetic defects. These genetic defects may not have an immediate effect on the child but will be passed on to following generations until other factors trigger abnormality.

So men who smoke may be harming themselves, their children, their grandchildren and great-grandchildren. This is a compelling reason to give up smoking now, long before trying to conceive a baby.

Researchers at the University of North Carolina, USA, analysed the histories of 15,000 children born between 1959 and 1966. They discovered that, when compared with children of non-smoking fathers, children of men smoking more than 20 cigarettes per day were:

- Twice as likely to suffer from a hare lip (cleft palate).
- Twice as likely to have a heart defect.
- Two and a half times more likely to have an abnormal narrowing of the urethra (tube through which urine is voided).

Another study looked at 220 children under the age of 14 suffering from childhood cancer. They discovered that, compared with children of non-smoking fathers, in the offspring of men who smoked tobacco (cigarettes, pipes or cigars) in the year before the children were born:

• Leukaemia was twice as common.
• Lymphoma (cancer of the lymph nodes) was twice as common.
• Brain cancer was 40 per cent more common.

When fathers smoked heavily (equivalent to eleven or more cigarettes per day) the relative risk of a child developing any childhood cancer was 70 per cent greater than that of children whose fathers did not smoke. The effect was even greater if the child was male.

Other studies suggest that fathers who smoke increase the risk of their offspring developing:

• Rhabdomyosarcoma (cancer of muscle).
• Neuroblastoma (cancer of the adrenal glands or sympathetic nervous system).

All these increased risks are partly because smoking cigarettes at least doubles the number of free radicals produced in the body every second – and we've already seen that 40 per cent of sperm damage is associated with free radical attack.

Fathers who continue to smoke while their partner is pregnant, and after the child is born, continue to increase the risk of their offspring dying young or developing a childhood cancer. Constituents of their tobacco smoke are absorbed passively by the pregnant mother and readily cross the placenta to the detriment of the foetus (see page 154).

These results have been confirmed time and again in the last 10 years since the first edition of this book. One study looked at the effects of paternal smoking, especially around the time of conception, in 642 children in China who developed cancer, and whose mothers were non-smokers, comparing them with a similar group of children who did not develop cancer. Paternal smoking around the time of conception was found to significantly increase the risk of childhood cancers, particularly acute leukaemia and lymphoma. The risks rose with the amount and duration of smoking for acute lymphocytic leukaemia, lymphoma and for all other cancers. Compared with children whose fathers had never smoked cigarettes, those whose fathers smoked more than five years prior to their conception were 3.8 times more likely to develop acute lymphocytic leukaemia, 4.5 times more likely to develop lymphoma and 2.7 times more likely to develop a brain tumour. Their overall risk of developing any cancer was 1.7 times greater than those whose fathers had not smoked. Statistically significant increased risks of cancer were restricted to children under the age of five at diagnosis or those whose fathers had smoked during all of the five years prior to conception.

The clear conclusion is that it is vital for a prospective father to stop smoking before starting his pre-conceptual programme and to remain non-smoking for the rest of his life – not just for his own health benefit, but for that of his future children and grandchildren.

Effect of vitamin C supplement on the sperm quality of smokers

Several reports indicate that men who smoke 20 or more cigarettes per day have blood vitamin C levels that are 20 per cent to 40 per cent lower than non-smokers. They also have reduced sperm counts, reduced sperm motility and increased risk of sperm abnormalities.

In one study, 75 men aged 20 to 35 years of age were given daily vitamin C supplements containing either none (placebo), 200 mg or 1,000 mg.

After four weeks, the group given 200 mg vitamin C per day showed an impressive 24 per cent improvement in sperm count, 18 per cent improvement in sperm motility and 24 per cent improvement in the number of sperm still viable after 24 hours. Improvement started just one week after supplementation.

In the group given daily supplements of 1,000 mg vitamin C, sperm count improved by 34 per cent, motility by 5 per cent and viability by 34 per cent. There were also significant improvements in other sperm quality factors such as lack of clumping together (agglutination), fewer abnormal forms and more sperm alive after 24 hours.

Results after taking supplements for four weeks are shown in the following table.

Improvement in six sperm qualities

Sperm qualities	200 mg vitamin C supplements	1,000 mg vitamin C supplements
Count	+24%	+34%
Motility	+18%	+5%
Viability	+24%	+34%
Agglutination	+13%	+67%
24 hour viability	+13%	+64%
Reduction in abnormal forms	+4%	+33%

The average improvement in the six sperm qualities after four weeks of supplementation was 15 per cent in men taking 200 mg vitamin C per day and a massive 40 per cent in men taking 1,000 mg per day. There was no significant change in the placebo group.

Further analysis showed that the positive effect of sperm quality was directly linked to the increased vitamin C levels present in both the men's blood and in their seminal fluid.

Men who smoke and men who are diabetic need twice as much vitamin C to neutralise the increased rate of damaging free radical reactions in their body. Vitamin C plays a dual role in protecting sperm (see page 209).

Cannabis and sperm

Cannabis resin and marijuana (dried leaves and flower tops) are derived from the hemp plant, cannabis sativa. Recreational use of these drugs is prohibited in many countries, but they remain widely available and widely used.

The active ingredient in cannabis and marijuana is tetrahydro-cannabinol (THC), a substance chemically related to our steroid hormones such as testosterone. As a result, tetrahydrocannabinol tends to accumulate in the testicles.

Heavy use of these illicit drugs (five to fifteen joints per week over six months) lowers the blood testosterone level and secondarily lowers the sperm count. More abnormal sperm are formed and those that are structurally normal tend to have decreased motility.

Even smoking just one joint can lower your testosterone level for over 36 hours. Drug use is also associated with lowered libido and an increased tendency to male impotence.

Use of all recreational as well as prescribed drugs should be avoided during the pre-conceptual care period.

Coffee and sperm

Some studies suggest that moderate intakes of caffeine can affect sperm motility, while large intakes can cause complete immobilisation.

Against this is the fact that a caffeine derivative, pentoxifylline, has been shown to increase the fertilising capacity of sperm during in-vitro (test tube) fertilisation studies. The caffeine derivative acts as a sort of turbo charge to sluggish sperm in some subfertile men. The effect is short-lasting but may provide enough boost to allow fertilisation to occur.

It's best to keep your intake of tea, coffee and caffeine-containing soft drinks to a minimum during the pre-conceptual care period but there's no need to avoid them altogether. A safe maximum would seem to be around three cups a day.

Diabetes and sperm

Until recently, anecdotal evidence suggested that diabetic men were less fertile than normal. There is now evidence that the opposite may be true.

Sperm analysis from seventeen insulin-dependent men and sixteen non-diabetic men showed that there were no differences in sperm track speed, path velocity, progressive velocity (speed from A to B) or lateral head displacement (tendency to swing head from side to side and so slow progress) between the two groups. Sperm from diabetic men, however, swam in much straighter lines.

Diabetics' sperm had a linearity (tendency to go in a straight line) of 70 per cent and a linear index of 84 per cent compared with 59 per cent and 76 per cent respectively for sperm from non-diabetic men. This suggests that a diabetic's sperm swim in a straighter line and get from A (e.g. cervix) to B (e.g. newly released egg) more quickly and on target than sperm from a non-diabetic man.

Chlamydia and sperm

Chlamydia trachmatis is one of the most common sexually transmissible diseases in the Western world. In men, this usually produces soreness and a burning discharge from the end of the penis known as NSU (non-specific urethritis).

Untreated chlamydia infection in women is associated with subfertility due to inflammation of the Fallopian tubes. It is now known that chlamydia infection decreases fertility in males too.

A study involving over 450 men found that those with chlamydia infection have a lower sperm count, lower sperm motility and a higher percentage of abnormal sperm than men who are free from the infection. After a 10-day course of antibiotics, those cured of the infection showed a significant improvement in semen quality compared with those in whom infection was not eradicated.

If you notice any unusual discharge, soreness or other symptoms which might indicate a sexually transmissible disease, it is important to attend a genito-urinary (special or GUM) clinic for a check-up early on during your pre-conceptual care programme.

Exercise and sperm

It is important to maintain a good level of fitness for general health. Vigorous exercise lasting for at least 20 to 30 minutes, three times per week, is recommended.

It is possible to overdo exercise, however. Strenuous exercise can cut sperm counts by half, according to a recent study. When fit men who trained regularly were asked to double their usual training programme to more than four days per week for two weeks, their sperm concentrations dropped by an amazing 43 per cent.

Three months later, their sperm counts had dropped even more, to 52 per cent lower than before they overtrained. Excessive training also increased the number of immature and non-viable sperm found in the semen.

The most likely explanation for these findings is a fall in testosterone levels that occurs immediately after exercising. This affects spermatogenesis for as long as several months later.

Hernia operations and sperm

Operations to repair inguinal (groin) or scrotal hernias may affect fertility. One survey of almost 600 men who had had inguinal hernia repairs found that one in eight had a wasted (atrophic) testicle on the operated side.

Semen quality in all hernia repair patients was markedly reduced, even when the testicles were normal. These effects were probably caused by too tight a repair or post-operative swelling subsequently restricting the blood supply to the testicle on that side. Another possibility is disruption of the normal blood-sperm barrier. If blood and sperm mix, anti-sperm antibodies may be produced. This will affect both testicles.

If a man who is considering fathering a child has had a hernia repair in the past, it may be worth requesting a semen analysis towards the end of the pre-conceptual care period, when sperm are present in peak numbers and peak health, to ensure there are no obvious abnormalities.

Mumps and sperm

Mumps is well known to affect the testes – with inflammation (orchitis) occurring in 25 per cent to 35 per cent of cases. Symptoms include swelling and severe pain in the affected testis along with a high temperature.

When this occurs before puberty, complete recovery is the rule. If it occurs after puberty, sperm production in the infected testicle is usually affected and the testicle may shrink. This is caused by degenerative changes occurring in the seminiferous tubules. As a result, there is a marked decrease in sperm quality and numbers from the affected testis.

Usually, mumps orchitis only affects one testicle and the overall sperm count is acceptable. Degenerative changes may be observed in the other, apparently unaffected testicle, however.

In a recent study, 72 young Israeli soldiers were assessed following mumps attacks. Nineteen of these suffered from a clinical mumps orchitis. Semen analysis was encouraging. While some men had higher than normal numbers of abnormal sperm and lower sperm motility, all the men who had suffered mumps orchitis had sperm that were considered within the fertile range. Interestingly, the researchers also found that men who smoked seemed more likely to develop mumps orchitis than men with mumps who did not smoke.

In conclusion, if a man has suffered from mumps or orchitis in the past, his chance of normal fertility is excellent. By following a normal pre-conceptual regime, his sperm quality is likely to improve in a similar way to that of men who have not suffered from mumps orchitis. Some ex-mumps sufferers may wish to have a confirmatory sperm count before trying to conceive.

HIV and sperm

Modern techniques allow HIV-positive men to father healthy children without increasing the risk of infecting an HIV-negative partner.

Semen is 'washed' to remove the infective fraction. The most motile sperm are then isolated and used to artificially inseminate the partner after inducing ovulation.

In a trial involving 29 couples, 59 insemination attempts resulted in 17 pregnancies in 15 women. Each woman required from one to five insemination attempts. None of the women became HIV positive and all babies were HIV negative at follow-ups ranging from six months to three years. It is estimated that the technique has only a 4 per cent risk of inseminating the mother with infected sperm such that she subsequently becomes HIV positive.

Abstinence and sperm

Latest research suggests that men can increase their chances of fathering a child by abstaining from ejaculation for seven to ten days before their partner's peak fertile time.

Traditional advice was to abstain for only three days as it was thought that sperm quality would deteriorate after this time. The new research shows that sperm counts and volume of ejaculate were significantly higher after seven days' abstinence whilst other variables such as motility, viability and percentage of abnormal forms stayed the same as after only three days' abstinence.

Aspiration of sperm

Men with low sperm counts despite pre-conceptual care, and those in whom reversal of vasectomy has produced poor results, have new hope thanks to a pioneering technique.

Semen can now be aspirated (drawn) from the epididymis (the convoluted tube between the testis and the vas deferens) and processed by spinning, washing and filtering to collect healthy sperm, however low the sperm count. The technique has so far been used to allow seven men with severe spinal injury (paralysis and impotence) to father children.

This technique is not yet widely available but should become standard in the near future.

Providing a semen sample

Being asked to provide a sperm sample can be embarrassing but prior knowledge is helpful. Semen analysis is:

- An essential first step in investigating subfertility.
- A useful test to have done as part of the male pre-conceptual care programme.

If there is no clinical reason for performing the test, you may find you have to pay for the semen analysis to be done privately.

You should refrain from ejaculation for at least three days prior to the investigation. Specimens are obtained by masturbation into a clean, dry sample jar. This must be examined 'hot' and you may be advised to deliver the specimen on hospital premises to ensure it is as fresh as possible. Sperm are then directly examined under the microscope.

Normal range

Sperm volume	2–4 ml on average
Sperm count	20–200 million per ml
Sperm motility	more than 40 per cent actively mobile
Abnormal forms	less than 40 per cent abnormal

Interpretation of results

Low sperm count, low sperm mobility or excessive abnormal forms suggest subfertility. This may be caused by:

- Previous mumps orchitis.
- Poor nutrition (lack of antioxidants).
- Drugs, alcohol or smoking.
- Excess local heat and electrostatic electricity.
- Previous or current infection of the vas deferens or testicle.
- Undescended testicles (cryptorchidism).

- Faulty development of the testes (germinal aplasia).
- Pituitary gland deficiency.
- Thyroid hormone deficiency.

18

General male health

Body weight

Overweight males are less fertile than normal-weight males for a
number of reasons:

- Fatty (adipose) tissue secretes oestrogen hormone, which
  counteracts the masculinising effects of testosterone. Men who
  were obese since before puberty tend to have smaller testicles,
  a smaller penis, a lower sperm count and reduced libido
  compared with normal-weight males.
- Increased body fat surrounding or overhanging the genitals
  raises scrotal temperature which in turn reduces fertility (see
  page 199).
- Increased body weight leads to general unfitness and easy
  tiring, making sexual intercourse less of a pleasure and more of
  a chore.
- Male obesity implies an unhealthy diet high in saturated fat,
  excess calories and probably low in fibre, minerals and
  vitamins. Alcohol intake may also be higher than normal. All
  these factors adversely influence fertility.

It is important for a prospective father to lose any excess fat during
the pre-conceptual care period. Adopt a healthy diet similar to that
of your female partner (see page 43).

The daily dietary energy requirements for men are provided

below. These are for men of average activity and are averages only. Half the male population will need fewer calories than those quoted and half will need more.

Your calorie intake also depends on your current weight, your level of activity and your metabolic rate. The heavier you are, the more calories you need to maintain this extra bulk.

Daily calorie requirements for males of average activity (Kcal/day)

Age	Calories
11–14	2,220
15–18	2,755
19–59	2,550
60–74	2,355
75 and over	2,100

The next table allows you to work out your ideal pre-conceptual weight according to your height. The weight range given is wide to take account of men who are naturally tall and thin as well as those who are squatter and more muscular.

You will already have a fair idea of whether you need to lose weight. Any excess flab is best lost during your pre-conceptual programme. The healthier you and your diet are, the healthier your sperm and future offspring will be. For information on why a healthy diet is important for the quality and quantity of your sperm, see page 207.

As a general rule, if you have excessive weight to lose, aim to eat between 500 and 1,000 kcals fewer per day than you actually need. You will obtain the additional energy by burning flab.

Cut back on snacks, pastries, cakes, biscuits, crisps, confectionery, puddings and alcohol. Replace these with fruit and low-calorie drinks. Put less food on your plate and try to eat smaller portions of everything. If you tend towards inactivity, increase your exercise levels to burn off extra fat more quickly.

Optimum body weight for males
(based on BMI* of 20–25 kg/m^2)

Height		Optimum body weight range	
Metres	*Feet*	*Kilograms*	*Stones and pounds*
1.40	4' 8"	39–49	6st 2lb–7st 9lb
1.47	4' 10"	43–53	6st 10lb–8st 6lb
1.50	4' 11"	45–56	7st 1lb–8st 11lb
1.52	5'	46–58	7st 4lb–9st 1lb
1.55	5' 1"	48–60	7st 7lb–9st 5lb
1.57	5' 2"	49–61	7st 10lb–9st 8lb
1.60	5' 3"	51–64	8st 1lb–10st
1.63	5' 4"	53–66	8st 5lb–10st 5lb
1.65	5' 5"	55–68	8st 8lb–10st 9lb
1.68	5' 6"	56–70	8st 12lb–11st
1.70	5' 7"	58–72	9st 1lb–11st 4lb
1.73	5' 8"	60–75	9st 6lb–11st 10lb
1.75	5' 9"	61–76	9st 9lb–12st
1.78	5' 10"	63–79	9st 13lb–12st 6lb
1.80	5' 11"	65–81	10st 3lb–12st 9lb
1.83	6'	67–83	10st 7lb–13st 1lb
1.85	6' 1"	69–85	10st 11lb–13st 5lb
1.88	6' 2"	71–88	11st 2lb–13st 12lb
1.90	6' 3"	72–90	11st 5lb–14st 2lb
1.93	6' 4"	75–93	11st 10lb–14st 8lb

*For an explanation of body mass index (BMI) see page 113.

PART III
Conception

19

Trying to conceive

Once you and your partner have followed a pre-conceptual care programme for at least three months – preferably six – you will feel ready to try for conception.

Your average chance of conceiving is at least 20 per cent per month and most of you will achieve your target within one year. One study showed that 38 per cent of non-smoking women conceive during their first menstrual cycle after stopping contraception, compared to only 28 per cent of women who smoke.

Fertility naturally declines with age, as can be seen from the following table:

Age of woman	Average time to pregnancy	Monthly chance of pregnancy with artificial insemination
25 years	2–3 months	11%
35 years	6 months or longer	6.5%

Your chances of success will have improved considerably, however, whatever your age, through following a healthy pre-conceptual diet and lifestyle.

The father's sperm are present in maximised quality and quantity, while the prospective mother is primed with nutrient vitamins and minerals. These factors will increase the chance of a healthy fertilised egg implanting and developing beyond 20 days.

The following pages look more closely at the process of fertilisation. You may want to go back to the beginning of this book and reread the sections on the female menstrual cycle and oogenesis before considering ovulation kits and the process of conception described below.

Myths

There are a surprising number of *misconceptions* regarding fertility. According to one survey of 1,000 adults of childbearing age:

- Almost 50 per cent of British men and 39 per cent of women believe a woman needs an orgasm to get pregnant (she doesn't).
- 57 per cent of women and 76 per cent of men did not know that a woman is most fertile in the middle of the menstrual cycle. Many didn't even know there was a fertile peak.
- 45 per cent of women are worried that long-term use of the Pill will affect their ability to conceive (it doesn't seem to).
- 17 per cent of women under the age of 24 did not know how to get pregnancy confirmed.
- 8 per cent of women and 11 per cent of men believe pregnancy will occur within the first month of trying.

Other common and misleading beliefs are that:

- You cannot get pregnant the first time you make love. *Wrong*.
- You cannot get pregnant from intercourse during menstruation. *Wrong* – unusual yet possible.
- Douching after intercourse prevents pregnancy. *Wrong*.
- Jumping up and down after intercourse prevents pregnancy. *Wrong*.
- The worst contraceptive Pills to miss are those in the middle of the packet. *Wrong* – missing Pills at the start and finish of each

pack, and therefore extending the length of the seven-day Pill-free interval is worse.

- You only have to use precautions the first time you make love in any one session. *Wrong*.
- Women over the age of 35 cannot get pregnant easily. *Wrong* – women are at their fertile peak around the age of 24 years old. While fertility does decrease with age, one in twelve children are now born to women over the age of 35 years.

How often should you make love?

Traditionally, couples were advised to make love every two or three days to maintain the male sperm count and to ensure an almost constant presence of sperm within the female tract. This was found to help maintain semen at a volume in excess of 2 ml, with at least 20 million sperm per ml, and with more than 60 per cent to 75 per cent motile sperm of a normal shape and size. Some research now suggests that a couple may be able to maximise the chance of successful conception if the male abstains from ejaculation for seven to 10 days before the female's most fertile time of the cycle. It was found that after seven days' abstinence, sperm count and semen volume were significantly greater than if the men abstained for only three days, while sperm motility, viability and the percentage of abnormal forms stayed the same. This may prove useful information for couples who have experienced difficulty in conceiving.

Interestingly, fertility experts have discovered that women usually ovulate at around 4 pm. The best time to make love may therefore be around lunchtime on the day ovulation is due. It may be worth going home at lunchtime for a rendezvous with your partner, or even taking the day off work around the time of ovulation.

Sex selection of offspring

If things are left to nature, 105 boys are born for every 100 girls, though a slightly higher rate of infant death among boys makes the proportions roughly equal. (Interestingly, more babies are conceived in November in Britain, USA, Austria, Belgium and Germany than in any other month – possibly related to the onset of long, dark winter nights. In Holland and Switzerland, the most popular month for conception is January, while in Sweden, more babies are conceived in August than in any other month.)

More than one in 10 babies is born to couples who have taken more than a year to become pregnant. Danish research involving 56,000 births suggests that women who have problems conceiving may be twice as likely to have a pre-term birth (before 37 weeks) or low-birth-weight baby, or to need a Caesarean section. The risks seem to be higher for women having a second or subsequent baby than for those having their first baby. The reasons are currently unknown.

Within each male primitive germ cell, there are 46 chromosomes arranged as 23 pairs. One of these pairs – the sex chromosomes – is unequal, consisting of a fat X (female) chromosome and a smaller Y (male) chromosome. The Y chromosome provides all the genetic information needed for the development of male sexual characteristics. In its absence, female sexual characteristics will occur.

During the special cell division (meiosis) which results in each sperm having only half the genetic material present in every other male body cell (see page 186), the sex chromosome pair is split. One product of the cell division will receive the X chromosome and one will receive the Y chromosome. Half a man's sperm are therefore Y sperm and the other half are X sperm.

The female's eggs only ever contain an X (female) chromosome. When a sperm containing a Y chromosome fertilises the egg, a boy (XY) is produced. When a sperm containing an X chromosome fertilises the egg, a girl (XX) is produced.

It is now possible to improve on nature's odds and increase your chances of a child of selected sex. Most methods rely on the physical and immunological differences between X and Y sperm.

Sperm containing the fatter X (female) chromosome are heavier and swim more slowly, sluggishly yet persistently than sperm containing a Y chromosome. As this chromosome is light, the Y sperm can swim faster but with less stamina and it tends to tire more easily. Other things being equal, the race for the egg is usually won by the swifter Y chromosome – hence the slight preponderance of boys born worldwide.

When vaginal fluids are more strongly acid (just before ovulation), the more resilient X sperm have the advantage. This was the basis for folklore tips on DIY sex selection. They have a slightly better chance of success than leaving things up to nature.

Scientific methods to separate sperm into X and Y fractions exploit their different weights and speeds. Either albumin filters, dyes or electrical charges are used. Isolated sperm fractions are then used for artificial insemination into the womb.

Varying success rates are claimed ranging from 50 per cent (expected!) to 80 per cent but results cannot be guaranteed. The results seem to be more reliable if a couple are trying for a girl.

In the filter method of sperm separation, a test tube containing a viscous solution of human albumin protein is used to act almost like a race track. Sperm are laid on top of the solution and male sperm, which are lighter and have a smaller surface area, drop to the bottom of the tube quicker than the larger, heavier female sperm.

American scientists have recently perfected a method of labelling sperm which is claimed to be reliable. The technique is called Flow Cytometric Cell Sorting Technology. It can produce semen fractions that contain 82 per cent X (female) sperm or 75 per cent Y (male) sperm.

These samples are enriched using a technique called FISH – fluorescence in situ hybridisation. This enables the numbers of X and Y sperm to be labelled and counted. All sperm in a semen sample are marked by adding a dye that fluoresces in ultraviolet light. The semen is then specially agitated so that it breaks up into droplets, each drop containing one sperm. Drops containing female sperm glow more brightly than male drops as they contain more genetic material (fat X chromosome compared to small Y chromosome).

Each drop is then electrically charged, male sperm are made positive and female sperm negative. As droplets pass electrically charged plates, they are separated according to their sex and the charge they carry.

At present, this technique is only licensed for medical use – for example, to reduce the risk of having a child with an hereditary, sex-linked disorder such as muscular dystrophy which affects only boys – and not for cosmetic (social) reasons. There are moves to allow sex selection of offspring (e.g. by sexing embryos) to balance a family (e.g. when a couple have only sons, for example). Ways of immunising against either X or Y sperm are being sought for the future but no method has yet been perfected.

DIY *tips for trying to conceive a girl*

- After menstruation, have frequent intercourse until at least 24 hours before ovulation. Then avoid sex until at least a week after ovulation (use an ovulation predictor kit or natural fertility methods).
- Douche the vagina with a mildly acidic solution just before having sex. The solution is made by dissolving 5 ml (one teaspoon) of white vinegar in a pint of sterile, distilled water.
- Try to avoid the woman having an orgasm as stimulated secretions increase vaginal alkalinity.
- Try to ejaculate just inside the vagina, where conditions are more acidic, rather than higher up.
- It is said that men who enjoy real ale are more likely to father daughters than men who prefer lager!

DIY *tips for trying to conceive a boy*

- Avoid intercourse during the four days just before ovulation. Plan to make love at or just after ovulation (use an ovulation predictor kit or natural fertility methods).
- Douche the vagina with a mildly alkaline solution just before having sex. The solution is made by dissolving 5 ml (one tea-spoon) of sodium bicarbonate in a pint of sterile, distilled water.
- Ideally, the woman should have an orgasm just before ejaculation as stimulated secretions increase vaginal alkalinity.
- Try to ejaculate deep inside the vagina, preferably against the cervix, where conditions are more alkaline.

Food *intake and sex of baby*

Interestingly, pregnant women carrying boys seem to need more energy and have a 10 per cent higher energy intake during pregnancy than those carrying girls. It is thought that a signal from the foetus (e.g. testosterone) may increase appetite and increase food intake in women carrying boys. A recent study found that pregnant women carrying a boy ate 8 per cent more protein, 9 per cent more carbohydrates, 11 per cent more animal fats and 15 per cent more vegetable fats than those carrying a girl.

Ovulation predictor kits

Ovulation predictor kits are a useful and accurate way to help you estimate your most fertile phase (see page 3). Knowing when ovulation is about to occur will maximise your chances of conception. Tests are simple to perform and take only three to five minutes to provide up to 99 per cent accurate results.

Ovulation predictor kits measure the amount of luteinising hormone (LH) in your urine. This is always present in small amounts, but suddenly increases in concentration on your most fertile day. This surge in LH is what triggers ovulation.

Most women ovulate twelve to 36 hours after the LH surge is detected. As the egg can only be fertilised for six to 24 hours after ovulation, by having intercourse on the day you detect the surge and the day after you are increasing your chances of success.

How to use an ovulation predictor kit

There are two main types of ovulation predictor kit available. One is more complicated to use than the other. Both methods are described below to help you choose which one you would prefer.

You need a clock or timer to complete the tests accurately. You will be checking your urine every day from around the middle of your cycle, when ovulation is most likely, until your LH surge is detected.

Count the *first* day of your last period as day 1 and count forward successive days after that.

Reagent method (e.g. First Response)

This is the type of test used by many GPs, hospitals and laboratories. It is 99 per cent accurate.

- If your menstrual cycle is usually between 23 and 32 days long, you need to start checking your urine for the LH surge every day from day 11 (day 1 = first day of bleeding during your last period).
- If your menstrual cycle is usually 22 days long, or shorter, start testing on day 7.
- If your menstrual cycle is usually 33 or more days long, start testing on day 17, but check with your doctor for advice as a very long cycle may mean you are not ovulating regularly.

To perform the test, collect a fresh sample of urine each morning as soon as you get out of bed. Collect the sample in the container provided and make sure you do the test within three hours of collection. If you can't test within three hours, cover the sample and refrigerate it for up to twelve hours. Allow it to reach room temperature before testing.

Try not to shake the sample, as you should only use urine from the top of the container. Using the filtered dropper provided, slowly draw up a sample of urine from the top of the container. Squeeze urine from the dropper into the powder-filled test tube provided until you reach the marked line. Gently swirl the urine and then leave to stand for three minutes.

After three minutes, the urine solution is poured from the test tube into a special test well – a hollow in the plastic insert that comes with your kit. A colourless test liquid is added to the urine solution in the well and you are then ready to read the test results.

Each kit contains a shade card showing a reference colour. This is often a light pink. If the colour result from your test is the same, or darker than the reference colour, the ovulation prediction test is positive. Today is the day of your peak LH surge – your most fertile time for making love.

If the test shade is white or much paler than the reference shade, test again on the next day and so on.

Often, the first day on which you test your urine (according to cycle length as above) will be your peak LH day.

One-step method (e.g. Clearplan One Step)

This method does not involve having to mix reagents and is specifically designed for home use. It is at least 98 per cent accurate. It involves a test wand which has an absorbent tip at one end and two result windows on the handle.

Work out which day you need to start using the kit according to your cycle length (see below).

The one-step test is ideally used on the first urine you pass in the morning. This has the highest concentration of hormones. If using it later in the day, make sure you have not urinated for at least four hours previously.

Cycle length	Start test this number of days after your last period started
21	5
22	5
23	6
24	7
25	8
26	9
27	10
28	11
29	12
30	13
31	14
32	15
33	16
34	17
35	18
36	19
37	20
38	21
39	22
40	23

Remove a test wand from its foil pack and take off the cap. Holding the wand downwards, insert the absorbent sampler tip into your urine stream as you pee. The test should be held in position for at least five seconds. Make sure the entire absorbent section is wet, but don't get any urine on the windows in the handle.

Remove the sampler from your urine stream and replace the cap while holding the test with the sampler tip still pointing down. You can now rest the test wand on a flat surface and leave it for five minutes before reading the result.

After five minutes, there should be a blue line in the smaller of the two windows. This proves that the test is complete and working properly.

Now look at the larger window. This will tell you how much LH is present in your urine. If the larger window is blank, or has only a pale blue line, lighter than the one in the small window, you have not yet begun your LH surge. Continue with daily testing. If the larger window contains a blue line similar to that in the small window, your LH surge has begun.

Anovulatory cycles

In approximately one out of every thirteen menstrual cycles women do not ovulate and therefore cannot become pregnant in that particular month. If, after five days of testing, the LH surge is not detectable, you are probably experiencing an anovulatory cycle (see page 5). Carry on testing for several more days in case this is an unusually long ovulatory cycle for you.

Don't worry unduly if you don't seem to ovulate during any one cycle – this is fairly common. If you don't seem to ovulate for two to three consecutive cycles, consult your doctor. By taking a blood test, your doctor will know whether or not you are ovulating. This is determined by measuring your blood progesterone level on day 21 of your next menstrual cycle (i.e. 21 days after the first day of your last period).

If you seem to be experiencing regular anovulatory cycles, don't despair. After further investigatory blood tests, you can usually be prescribed a fertility drug to kick-start ovarian follicular maturation.

Ovulation can also be predicted using Calista to assess saliva (see page 19).

Ovulation predictor kits and contraception

Please note that if you are using the ovulation predictor kit to assist natural fertility methods of contraception, it's important to abstain from intercourse, or use a barrier method of contraception, during the fertile phase of your cycle (see page 16).

Sperm can survive in the female tract for several days and intercourse before ovulation can still result in fertilisation. You should not rely on unprotected intercourse until the second, absolutely infertile phase of your cycle has begun. This starts 48 hours after ovulation.

Ovulation does not occur until twelve to 36 hours after the ovulation predictor kit has detected your LH surge. Therefore, the second infertile phase of your cycle will not start until at least 36 plus 48 hours (84 hours) after the LH surge test is positive. Use other natural indicators of fertility to augment the ovulation predictor kit when using it to assist contraception during your pre-conceptual programme.

Short gaps between pregnancies

Women who leave a very short gap between pregnancies seem to be at increased risk of premature birth, low-birth-weight babies and neonatal death, according to a study involving 89,000 women having their second baby in Scotland. Those who had an interval of less than six months between pregnancies were more likely to have an extremely pre-term birth, a moderately pre-term birth, and to suffer a neonatal death not due to congenital abnormality. It is therefore worth leaving at least six months between pregnancies if you can – especially if the preceding pregnancy was associated with maternal or neonatal problems where the risks appeared to be greater. Latest research suggests a gap of three to five years between babies is optimal.

Conception

The modern view of conception is that it is a complex process. It starts with the fusion of a sperm and an egg but is not complete until implantation has occurred. Implantation itself is not considered complete until a functional placenta develops.

Studies suggest that implantation of a fertilised egg fails in at least 30 per cent of cases. Some failures to implant may be caused by genetic abnormalities in the fertilised egg – derived either from the maternal or the paternal chromosomes. Other failures may be caused by inhospitable conditions in the potential mother (e.g. high alcohol intake, low zinc levels, obesity, vitamin deficiency, systemic illness – see page 260).

The aim of pre-conceptual care is to improve the chances of successful implantation, a healthy pregnancy and finally, a perfect baby.

Conception stage 1: fertilisation

Fertilisation occurs when the egg fuses with a sperm. This usually happens in the upper one third of the Fallopian tube.

It's now thought that the egg plays an active role in fertilisation. Rather than waiting passively for sperm to reach it as it gently progresses down the tube, the egg releases an attractant chemical which entices sperm towards it. Different eggs, even from the same woman, seem to secrete varying amounts of this chemical and have varying success in attracting sperm.

Semen is initially thick and sticky after ejaculation. Within 20 to 30 minutes it liquefies because of the action of enzymes and the great sperm race begins. Some active sperm reach the Fallopian tubes within five minutes of deposition in the vagina. Others remain in the cervical mucus plug for several days, with a constant stream swimming up into the uterus and tubes.

On average, it takes around 70 minutes to reach the upper Fallopian tube once the sperm has left the cervical mucus plug. Only around 150 sperm out of the hundreds of millions ejaculated will reach the upper Fallopian tube at any one time to greet the descending egg.

Most of these become stuck to the outer coating (zona pellucida) of the egg. The sperm bind to this layer by a reaction between sperm receptors on the egg and a specific egg-binding protein on the sperm head. Binding of the sperm to the egg triggers release of enzymes found in a sac (acrosome) at the front of the sperm head. These enzymes dissolve the egg coating. Once a sperm penetrates the outer shell of the egg (zona pellucida) and reaches the egg's outer membrane, it fuses with it.

This triggers an electro-chemical reaction across the egg membrane which prevents other sperm from following suit. This reaction also changes the outer egg shell, hardening it as further protection against more than one sperm entering.

Sperm entry also triggers the final meiotic division of the egg and the second polar body is extruded (see page 8).

When the nucleus of the sperm fuses with that of the egg, 23 chromosomes in each combine to form a cell with 46 chromosomes and embryonic development begins. The newly fertilised egg divides repeatedly as it passes down the Fallopian tube to form a ball of cells.

Fluid accumulates inside to form a hollow bag of cells known as the blastocyst. This starts to implant in the receptive uterine lining (endometrium) approximately three to five days after fertilisation. By this time, the embryo consists of around sixteen cells.

Conception stage 2: implantation

While floating freely within the uterine cavity, the blastocyst receives nourishment and oxygen from the secretions of the endometrial glands.

Once the blastocyst comes into contact with the womb lining, it becomes attached and triggers a local increase in blood flow to that part of the endometrium.

Uterine blood vessels surrounding the blastocyst attachment site become more permeable and leak increasing amounts of nutrient plasma into the area. This is caused by substances secreted by the uterus (platelet activating factor; prostaglandins) and by the developing blastocyst itself (prostaglandins). The result is a rapid local swelling (oedema) around the site of implantation.

Within 24 hours of attachment, the blastocyst sends out tiny fingers of tissue which burrow between maternal endometrial cells to form an anchorage. The blastocyst secretes protein-digesting enzymes (proteases) and begins eroding a hollow for itself. Endometrial cells in the immediate vicinity start to break down, allowing the blastocyst to burrow deeper. This usually occurs between the fifth and ninth days after ovulation. The implantation site is usually on the upper back wall of the uterus, near the midline, but this is not invariable.

As the blastocyst burrows into the uterus, slight bleeding occurs. A fine balance between local chemicals encouraging blood to clot and those causing clots to dissolve (fibrinolytic agents) is set up.

In humans, altered blood clotting mechanisms seem to be a common feature among women who suffer recurrent spontaneous abortions for no obvious reason.

Implantation bleeding can be heavy enough for the new mother to notice as a pinkish discharge or may even simulate a light period. This is frequently mistaken for the beginning of the next menstruation that would usually be expected around this time.

Once pregnancy is eventually diagnosed, this false period makes early calculation of the date of delivery wrong by up to a month.

Formation of the deciduas

As the blastocyst burrows in, cells on the surface of the endometrium increase their content of sugar stores (glycogen) and fat (lipid). They also increase their protein output and their connections with surrounding cells.

These changes are part of the so-called decidua reaction. Initially, this reaction occurs around the site of implantation, but later extends to the entire lining of the womb. Its purpose is not fully understood, but the formation of a decidua may:

- Help nourish the developing embryo.
- Protect maternal tissues from extensive erosion by the blastocyst.

- Isolate multiple embryos to ensure the development of each independently of failure at adjacent implantation sites.
- Protect the embryo against immunological rejection by the mother.
- Provide structural support for the embryo.
- Secrete certain hormones.

It's also thought that the developing foetus is able to absorb and use the nutrients released as endometrial cells break down to allow implantation.

Successful implantation

By the eleventh or twelfth day after ovulation, the products of conception have sunk beneath the surface of the endometrium and are now completely embedded. The surface hole in the endometrium through which the blastocyst eroded becomes plugged by a blood clot and later closes completely.

The placenta starts to develop and acts as a go-between for the maternal circulation and that of the developing foetus. Conception has now medically and legally occurred.

The developing placenta secretes a hormone, human chorionic gonadotrophin (HCG), which acts as a signal to the corpus luteum (see page 5) that successful implantation has occurred. The corpus luteum then persists until about the fourth month of pregnancy instead of deteriorating. It continues to secrete oestrogen and high levels of progesterone. These are essential to maintain a thick endometrium and prevent menstruation during early pregnancy.

The placenta slowly takes over this hormone-producing role and from around six weeks' gestation could secrete enough hormones to maintain pregnancy itself should anything happen to the corpus.

The HCG secreted by the developing placenta also forms the basis for modern sensitive pregnancy tests (see page 246).

The foetus as a transplant

The mother and foetus are two genetically distinct human beings with different surface cell markers. In effect, the foetus is equivalent to a transplanted foreign tissue in which perhaps half of the surface 'identity' markers are the same as the mother's own.

For some reason no one yet understands, this foetal transplant is tolerated and rejection rarely occurs. It may be that identity antigens (proteins that trigger an immune response) are not expressed on the parts of the placenta that are in close contact with maternal tissues. Another theory is that the hundreds of millions of sperm produced during each ejaculation play a role. They may overwhelm the mother's immune system within the Fallopian tubes. As the combined sperm will contain the same genetic markers the foetus has received from its father, the sperm may somehow induce a tolerance to these.

The hormone progesterone also plays a role. Research has shown that progesterone can inhibit parts of the immune system (T-cell-mediated responses) which are involved in tissue rejection. As progesterone also damps down contraction of the uterus, this hormone is important in preventing early miscarriage.

Latest research shows that the developing blastocyst itself also secretes a soluble substance which interferes with the way immune cells (lymphocytes) proliferate. These soluble substances are present at the time of implantation and damp down local immune responses. This may help to explain the establishment of maternal tolerance towards the genetically different foetus.

Early diagnosis of pregnancy

Fertilisation usually occurs in the middle of the menstrual cycle. By the time your period is one day overdue, you may already be two weeks pregnant.

Pregnancy tests

As the placenta develops, it secretes a hormone called human chorionic gonadotrophin (HCG). This is a glycoprotein – a mixture

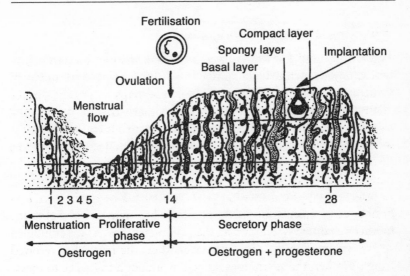

Fertilisation

Compact layer

Spongy layer

Implantation

Basal layer

Ovulation

Menstrual
flow

1 2 3 4 5 14 28

Menstruation | Proliferative phase | Secretory phase

Oestrogen | Oestrogen + progesterone

Hormone levels during normal pregnancy

of lactose (milk sugar) and protein – which is detectable in blood as early as 48 hours after conception and in the urine 72 hours after conception.

Modern pregnancy tests are remarkably accurate. Use a home kit or take a sample of early morning urine to a pharmacist. This can be done from the first day of a missed period as it will already be two weeks after fertilisation of the egg. It's best to use the first specimen of urine you pass in the morning as this will contain the highest concentration of the pregnancy test hormone HCG.

A positive pregnancy test is almost always correct but as at least 30 per cent of fertilised eggs fail to develop beyond the first 20 days, a period may start and the test subsequently prove negative. This is obviously quite distressing if a woman has had difficulty conceiving in the past.

Negative results can sometimes occur even though you are pregnant. Wait a week and, if your period still hasn't occurred, repeat the test. If it is still negative, consult your doctor as soon as possible.

Symptoms and signs of pregnancy

The corpus luteum in the ovary secretes large amounts of oestrogen and progesterone, which contribute to the symptoms of early pregnancy.

Some women seem to know intuitively that they are pregnant without being able to explain why. Others suffer pronounced morning sickness while many mothers bloom with no ill effects at all. The common early symptoms and signs of pregnancy are:

- A missed period or an unusually light period.
- Nausea and sometimes vomiting.
- Breast changes:
  - tingling;
  - tenderness;
  - distension of superficial veins;
  - darkening of the nipples.
- Needing to pass water more frequently – possibly in the night.
- A tendency towards constipation.
- Feeling increasingly tired.
- Having a strange, metallic taste in your mouth.
- Going off certain foods.
- Craving other foods.
- Increased blood flow to the genitals causing:
  - increased vaginal discharge;
  - a bluish tinge to the vagina;
  - softening of the cervix.

A doctor can often detect early vaginal and cervical changes but internal examinations at this time are not popular. If a spontaneous miscarriage were to occur, the woman may feel the examination was to blame.

The following obstetric chart lets you estimate the date your baby is due. Go to the date on which your last menstrual period *started* (top line). Underneath this is your estimated date of delivery, assuming a normal gestation time.

Top figure (bold) = date of last menstrual period (LMP)

Bottom figure (light) = expected date of delivery (EDD)

LMP	1	2	3	4	5	6	7	8	9	10	11	12	13	14	15	16	17	18	19	20	21	22	23	24	25	26	27	28	29	30	31	→
Jan	1	2	3	4	5	6	7	8	9	10	11	12	13	14	15	16	17	18	19	20	21	22	23	24	25	26	27	28	29	30	31	**Jan**
Oct	8	9	10	11	12	13	14	15	16	17	18	19	20	21	22	23	24	25	26	27	28	29	30	31	1	2	3	4	5	6	7	Nov
Feb	1	2	3	4	5	6	7	8	9	10	11	12	13	14	15	16	17	18	19	20	21	22	23	24	25	26	27	28				**Feb**
Nov	8	9	10	11	12	13	14	15	16	17	18	19	20	21	22	23	24	25	26	27	28	29	30	1	2	3	4	5				Dec
Mar	1	2	3	4	5	6	7	8	9	10	11	12	13	14	15	16	17	18	19	20	21	22	23	24	25	26	27	28	29	30	31	**Mar**
Dec	6	7	8	9	10	11	12	13	14	15	16	17	18	19	20	21	22	23	24	25	26	27	28	29	30	31	1	2	3	4	5	Jan
Apr	1	2	3	4	5	6	7	8	9	10	11	12	13	14	15	16	17	18	19	20	21	22	23	24	25	26	27	28	29	30		**Apr**
Jan	6	7	8	9	10	11	12	13	14	15	16	17	18	19	20	21	22	23	24	25	26	27	28	29	30	31	1	2	3	4		Feb
May	1	2	3	4	5	6	7	8	9	10	11	12	13	14	15	16	17	18	19	20	21	22	23	24	25	26	27	28	29	30	31	**May**
Feb	5	6	7	8	9	10	11	12	13	14	15	16	17	18	19	20	21	22	23	24	25	26	27	28	1	2	3	4	5	6		Mar
June	1	2	3	4	5	6	7	8	9	10	11	12	13	14	15	16	17	18	19	20	21	22	23	24	25	26	27	28	29	30		**June**
Mar	8	9	10	11	12	13	14	15	16	17	18	19	20	21	22	23	24	25	26	27	28	29	30	31	1	2	3	4	5	6		Apr
Jul	1	2	3	4	5	6	7	8	9	10	11	12	13	14	15	16	17	18	19	20	21	22	23	24	25	26	27	28	29	30	31	**Jul**
Apr	7	8	9	10	11	12	13	14	15	16	17	18	19	20	21	22	23	24	25	26	27	28	29	30	1	2	3	4	5	6	7	May
Aug	1	2	3	4	5	6	7	8	9	10	11	12	13	14	15	16	17	18	19	20	21	22	23	24	25	26	27	28	29	30	31	**Aug**
May	8	9	10	11	12	13	14	15	16	17	18	19	20	21	22	23	24	25	26	27	28	29	30	31	1	2	3	4	5	6	7	June
Sept	1	2	3	4	5	6	7	8	9	10	11	12	13	14	15	16	17	18	19	20	21	22	23	24	25	26	27	28	29	30		**Sept**
June	8	9	10	11	12	13	14	15	16	17	18	19	20	21	22	23	24	25	26	27	28	29	30	1	2	3	4	5	6	7		Jul
Oct	1	2	3	4	5	6	7	8	9	10	11	12	13	14	15	16	17	18	19	20	21	22	23	24	25	26	27	28	29	30	31	**Oct**
July	8	9	10	11	12	13	14	15	16	17	18	19	20	21	22	23	24	25	26	27	28	29	30	31	1	2	3	4	5	6	7	Aug
Nov	1	2	3	4	5	6	7	8	9	10	11	12	13	14	15	16	17	18	19	20	21	22	23	24	25	26	27	28	29	30		**Nov**
Aug	8	9	10	11	12	13	14	15	16	17	18	19	20	21	22	23	24	25	26	27	28	29	30	31	1	2	3	4	5	6		Sept
Dec	1	2	3	4	5	6	7	8	9	10	11	12	13	14	15	16	17	18	19	20	21	22	23	24	25	26	27	28	29	30	31	**Dec**
Sept	8	9	10	11	12	13	14	15	16	17	18	19	20	21	22	23	24	25	26	27	28	29	30	31	1	2	3	4	5	6	7	Oct

Sexual activity during pregnancy

It is commonly believed that sexual intercourse during pregnancy can lead to miscarriage or premature rupturing of membranes with pre-term delivery. There is some truth in this, but risks are probably not significant.

Throughout early pregnancy – three to five months – couples may safely make love, unless the woman has suffered a miscarriage in the past. If a threatened miscarriage occurs, with spotting of blood and/or low abdominal cramps, sex should be avoided as a precautionary measure. Follow the advice of your doctor.

A study in the USA looked at 588 women who had experienced a pre-term delivery or premature rupturing of membranes. All were questioned on the type and frequency of their sexual experience: position during intercourse, kissing on the mouth and occurrence of orgasm, with or without penetrative sex.

Making love with the woman on top or with the side-to-side position (vaginal entry from the rear) did not have any bearing on pregnancy outcome. It was found, however, that the missionary position (man on top) for making love was associated with an increased risk of pre-term labour with or without premature rupturing of membranes.

The relative risks of sexual activity in late pregnancy (1.9 to 1) are probably not great compared to the increased risks associated with exposure to cigarette smoke (relative risk of 4.2 to 1).

It is therefore more important for a pregnant woman to avoid exposure to cigarette smoke than to curtail her conjugal pleasures. Certainly a woman should not go out of her way to avoid having an orgasm.

Women who have a past history of pre-term labour or previous cervical surgery are usually advised caution during any sexual intercourse occurring after the sixth month of pregnancy.

Simple tips for making love during pregnancy:

• Have gentle rather than rough sex.
• Woman on top, or side-to-side rear entry, is safest.

- The man should avoid giving oral sex to the pregnant woman (cunnilingus). This has rarely been associated with an air embolus – air entering the bloodstream through the expanded uterine blood lakes occurring during pregnancy.
- If intercourse hurts, or you notice any blood loss, stop and seek medical advice.

20

Antenatal tests

Antenatal care is designed to elicit risk factors in pregnancy and to monitor foetal development. Listening to the foetal heart, counting foetal movements and measuring expansion of the womb are all simple tests of well-being.

Ultrasound scan

Ultrasound involves passing high-frequency sound waves through the body, which bounce back from tissues of different density in different ways. Returning signals are analysed by computer and translated into a visual image. This allows direct examination of the foetus through the abdominal wall or occasionally through the vagina.

Scanning measures foetal length, girth and head diameter to assess age, locates the placenta and diagnoses anatomical abnormalities such as spina bifida, cleft lip, cystic kidneys, abnormal brain structure, etc. Sex can sometimes be predicted but not always reliably.

Recently, the safety of repeated ultrasound scans was called into question. A study of 2,834 women was undertaken in the hope of proving that routine ultrasound testing improved pregnancy outcome. Its results suggested the opposite.

Although ultrasound was useful for screening against malformations and assessing gestational age, it did not significantly improve pregnancy outcome.

Those pregnancies in which ultrasound testing was repeatedly performed, at 18, 24, 28, 34 and 38 weeks, were more likely to have babies of low weight (less than 30 per cent for their gestational age) compared with babies who were only exposed to ultrasound testing at 18 weeks.

These findings may be a chance statistical finding, but further investigation is essential. In the meantime, it is important to remember that ultrasound scanning can detect physical congenital abnormalities at an early stage in pregnancy.

Another recent study suggested that babies who are scanned by ultrasound are more likely to be left-handed than babies who are not scanned. Out of 1,335 eight-year-olds studied in Norway, 7 per cent of those who received antenatal ultrasound screening were left-handed compared with 5 per cent not screened. In addition, 19 per cent of those screened were classed as ambidextrous compared with 15 per cent of those unscreened.

The researchers claim that ultrasound scanning may influence brain development at 16 to 22 weeks. Other specialists are sceptical, saying that the study was too small to be significant and that eight years of age is too young to assess which hand is dominant.

Detecting Down's syndrome

Every woman who discovers she is pregnant hopes to give birth to a healthy, normal child. Sadly, however, one in 20 babies is born with a congenital malformation and - although the vast majority are relatively minor - a major abnormality is diagnosed in around 1 per cent of pregnancies. The risk of chromosomal abnormalities increases dramatically with age and, with more women now postponing childbirth until their thirties or beyond, the level of maternal anxiety is inevitably increased.

Blood tests to screen for Down's syndrome in early pregnancy are routinely offered in most regions. These tests measure the level of a number of different blood chemicals such as alpha-feto protein and beta-HCG. The results are assessed depending on maternal age and the gestational age of the pregnancy. Ultrasound testing can also predict Down's syndrome using a technique known as nuchal translucency screening.

Nuchal translucency screening is carried out between the 11th and 14th weeks of pregnancy to measure the amount of fluid behind the foetal neck. The nuchal translucency is detected on ultrasound as a black space between the cervical spine and over-lying foetal skin. If the width of the nuchal translucency is increased (e.g. above the 99th centile of 3.5 mm) there is an increased risk of the foetus having an abnormal number of chromosomes, a genetic syndrome or a structural abnormality such as a major heart defect. Why these conditions increase the nuchal translucency is unknown, but it may be linked with fluid accumulation during heart failure or alterations in lymphatic drainage.

Nuchal translucency screening can predict 78 per cent of foetal chromosomal abnormalities for a false positive rate of 4.7 per cent. This does, of course, mean that even when the test is 'normal' there is still a 22 per cent chance of an undetected chromosomal abnormality, and that where the nuchal translucency is high, the baby may well be perfectly healthy. Counselling is therefore vitally important, with each couple receiving all the time they need to discuss the statistics and the full implications of their results.

If you are pregnant and concerned about your risk of conceiving a child with a foetal abnormality, it is important to discuss this with your GP or consultant as early as possible.

If blood tests or nuchal translucency screening suggest an increased risk of Down's syndrome, the mother is offered amnio-centesis for a definite diagnosis.

Amniocentesis

Amniocentesis entails inserting a fine needle through the mother's abdomen and collecting a sample of amniotic fluid. This can be done from around 14 to 16 weeks' gestation and allows direct genetic examination of foetal cells and examination of paired chromosomes.

Amniocentesis can detect genetic abnormalities such as absent or additional chromosomes, e.g. Trisomy 21.

Amniocentesis can accurately determine a baby's gender by identifying whether the two sex chromosomes are present as XX (girl) or XY (boy). This is useful in predicting inherited sex-linked conditions such as Duchenne's Dystrophy.

Amniocentesis does carry a small risk of miscarriage (0.5 per cent to 1 per cent) and cannot safely be performed before 16 weeks. It may also adversely affect foetal lung development.

Chorionic villus sampling

This tests for the same conditions as amniocentesis by biopsying small amounts of tissue from the placenta. This is done as early as eight weeks of pregnancy but carries a 1 per cent to 2 per cent risk of miscarriage. There is also a risk of damaging the early foetal vascular system (arteries and veins).

Embryoscopy

Embryoscopy involves viewing the embryo directly from five weeks' gestation via an endoscope passed through the cervix.

This picks up a range of genetic syndromes too subtle to be identified by transvaginal ultrasound at such an early stage. The advantage of this procedure over tests performed later, at 16 weeks, is that if a therapeutic abortion is requested, termination is much less traumatic for all concerned.

There is a small risk of miscarriage with embryoscopy – comparable to that of amniocentesis – of 0.5 to 1 per cent. This technique provides an access route for future gene therapy.

At present, the only human tissue that can be used for cell transfer into an embryo is bone marrow. Many ethical and legal considerations need to be addressed before the full potential of embryoscopy is realised.

Termination of pregnancy

Sadly, the decision to terminate a pregnancy sometimes has to be made. It is important to know that any surgical procedure involving the uterus (e.g. insertion of a contraceptive coil, termination of pregnancy) carries a small risk of complications such as acute infection, chronic pelvic inflammatory disease and perforation of the womb.

Despite this, new evidence suggests that women who have previously had a termination need not worry unduly that their future fertility will be affected. Women who had unplanned pregnancies between 1976 and 1987 were followed up for several years. Of these, 433 elected to have a termination, while 1,035 continued with the pregnancy. Follow-up showed that there was no significant difference in the time these women took to become pregnant again in the future.

Another study involving 9,299 women also found no reduction in future fertility among those who had previously had a termination.

21

Miscarriage

Miscarriage, also known medically as a spontaneous abortion, is defined as the early failure of pregnancy before the 24th week of gestation. After this time, the sad occasion of foetal death is classified as a stillbirth.

Between 20 and 80 per cent of newly fertilised eggs (zygotes) fail to implant in the uterine wall. This is known as pre-implantation wastage and occurs before conception is medically or legally recognised.

Of those zygotes that do successfully implant and start to produce a placenta, around 30 per cent miscarry – most before the mother is even aware she is pregnant. The next period may be slightly later and slightly heavier than usual, but that is all.

Sadly, of all pregnancies that are recognised as such by the mother, approximately 15 per cent fail to continue beyond the first five months of gestation. Twice as many will threaten to miscarry, with spotting of blood and/or period-like abdominal pains.

After a mother has had one miscarriage, her risk of another is twice that of a woman who has not previously had a miscarriage. After two consecutive miscarriages, the risk increases so that around 30 per cent of future pregnancies miscarry. This still means there is a 70 per cent chance of a pregnancy continuing to successful delivery of a child.

The risks do not continue to increase with each subsequent miscarriage, even though it may feel like it to a couple who have suffered through six or more miscarriages, one after the other. The future chance of a successful pregnancy still remains at around 50 per cent unless a specific, recurrent abnormality is diagnosed. In this case, your own physician can give you a more accurate assessment of your chances.

Genetic causes of miscarriage

The vast majority of miscarriages are due to a one-off genetic disorder of the egg or sperm which makes the continued development of the fertilised egg impossible.

Usually, the special cell division (meiosis) resulting in each sperm or egg having only half the genetic information of other body cells (i.e. 23 chromosomes instead of 46) goes wrong.

The egg or sperm may lack some vital genetic information, or, more commonly, an extra chromosome or set of chromosomes is present. This often occurs immediately after fertilisation when the second polar body fails to leave the fertilised egg (see page 8).

Research shows that chromosomal abnormalities are detected in up to 60 per cent of recognised miscarriages, 5 per cent of stillbirths and 0.5 per cent of all live births. These figures suggest that around 10 per cent of all recognised pregnancies (half of spontaneous miscarriages) are identified as genetically abnormal.

These genetic accidents are usually just that – an accident, possibly induced in a single germ cell by free radical attack (see page 101), toxins or exposure to irradiation. Only if the condition is an hereditary one will the risk of recurrent miscarriage increase.

Chromosomal abnormalities are not always incompatible with reproduction. Several recognised syndromes exist in which parts of chromosomes are missing or present in excessive numbers (see below).

It's estimated that one in every 20 babies is born with a congenital malformation and that 5 per cent of the population suffer from a genetic disorder.

Most infants with birth defects are born to women with no obvious risk factors, so detection of future problems is not always possible during the pre-conceptual care period.

Increasing maternal age

It is natural for the risk of a miscarriage to increase as you get older. Research suggests the risk of miscarriage doubles between the twenties and early thirties, then doubles again between the early and late thirties. This is caused by the increasing age of maternal egg follicles, which have been present in the female ovaries since birth. As well as increasing the risk of miscarriage, increasing maternal age is also linked with the risk of producing a child with genetic disorder.

Down's syndrome, for example, occurs when an extra chromosome 21 is present in foetal cells (Trisomy 21). The following table gives the estimated risk of having a child with Down's syndrome according to maternal age.

Mother's age	Risks of a child with Down's syndrome
28	1 in 1,000
30	1 in 880
32	1 in 720
34	1 in 460
36	1 in 280
38	1 in 180
40	1 in 100
42	1 in 70
44	1 in 40
46	1 in 25
48	1 in 15
50	1 in 10

Pre-conceptual care is especially important for women over the age of 35. Ensuring an adequate intake of antioxidant vitamins and minerals throughout life, but especially during the pre-conceptual care period, will help keep your risk of spontaneous genetic mutations to a minimum.

Women over the age of 35, and those who have previously had an affected child, are offered techniques that exclude genetic abnormalities in future pregnancies. These include amniocentesis (aspiration of amniotic fluid to examine sloughed foetal cells) and chorionic villus sampling (removal of a small piece of placental tissue for analysis).

Non-genetic causes of miscarriage

Of the 40 per cent to 50 per cent of miscarriages that are not caused by a genetic abnormality, many are of uncertain origin. The foetus starts to develop normally but then, because of some physical insult or deficiency, becomes deformed or is rendered incapable of further development. Possible causes include:

- Smoking.
- Nutritional deficiency of a vitamin or mineral.
- Bacterial or viral infection.
- Hormonal imbalance.
- Pre-existing maternal disease.
- Maternal disease associated with pregnancy itself.
- Maternal anatomical abnormalities.
- Immunological incompatibility between the foetus and the mother.
- Altered blood clotting mechanisms (see page 244).
- Drugs, including alcohol.

Some of these are discussed briefly below to show how pre-conceptual care can be important, especially if you have suffered a miscarriage in the past.

Nutritional deficiency

Deficiency of all nutrients, but especially of the B group vitamins, folate, essential fatty acids, calcium, magnesium and zinc, is associated with an increased risk of subfertility and early miscarriage. Lack of these nutrients interferes with cell division and DNA replication, a process occurring at a tremendous rate during foetal development.

Smoking

Women who smoke have a 27 per cent higher chance of suffering a miscarriage than non-smokers. Even passive smoking, especially where the mother lives with a smoker, has been linked with 4,000 miscarriages per year in the UK (see page 154).

Bacterial or viral infections

Diseases such as rubella, chlamydia, anaerobic vaginosis, cyto-megalovirus, etc. can result in miscarriage or congenital deformity if contracted during early pregnancy (see page 133).

Other infections, such as influenza, pneumonia, appendicitis, etc. can also trigger miscarriage, especially during the first three months of pregnancy. This may be a mechanism to protect the mother, whose immune system is naturally depressed during pregnancy, thereby interfering with her ability to fight infection.

As physical stress increases the body's needs for many vitamins and minerals, intercurrent infections also induce a relative nutrient deficiency, especially in chronic (long-term) grumbling types of infection, e.g. acute cystitis, vaginal bacterial imbalance. This can also trigger miscarriage.

Hormonal imbalance

There is less certainty regarding miscarriage and hormonal imbalance. Some researchers believe an inadequate corpus luteum (the collapsed follicle from which the egg was recently released) is at fault.

Early pregnancies can only continue developing if supported by high levels of progesterone hormone secreted by the corpus luteum. Basically, progesterone is needed to prevent shedding of the endo-metrium (womb lining) when the next period is due. Progesterone is also needed to suppress maternal immunity so that the foreign foetal tissue is not rejected.

The corpus luteum is maintained by a hormone signal (HCG – human chronic gonadotrophin) secreted by the developing placenta. Failure of the corpus luteum may occur because of a lack of sensitivity to HCG, or an innate inability to secrete enough progesterone.

In some countries, e.g. France, USA, progesterone injections or suppositories are given after ovulation (i.e. pre-conception) and throughout early pregnancy in women suffering repeated miscarriages. This may increase their chances of a successful outcome, but is not universally accepted as an effective treatment.

Another hormone imbalance linked with early miscarriage is a high level of luteinising hormone (LH). This seems to alter egg maturation before it is released from the ovary, making future miscarriage more likely. Treatment with the drug buserelin, which works by suppressing secretion of FSH and LH from the pituitary gland, may help.

Pre-existing maternal disease

Some common medical conditions such as diabetes mellitus (see page 129), high blood pressure (see page 129), thyroid problems and anaemia increase the risk of miscarriage if not carefully monitored and controlled. If you suffer from any of these conditions, consult your doctor before conception so your care can be planned.

Auto-immune disease: SLE

In auto-immune diseases, an overactive immune system makes antibodies against normal body structures. In some cases, these antibodies attack the placenta or foetus as well.

SLE is the auto-immune disease most usually linked with miscarriage – 25 per cent of sufferers have difficulty carrying pregnancy to term. Treatment with high-dose steroids and low-dose aspirin (to damp down the effects of the disease) is needed, starting during the pre-conceptual care period.

The best time for a woman with SLE to become pregnant is when the disease has been in remission for at least six months. Some women also require a drug called azathioprine to modify their immune response. This drug seems to be safe during pregnancy.

Women with SLE tend to have high levels of anti-phospholipid antibody, aimed against cell membranes. These are also present in 15 per cent of women suffering a miscarriage for no known cause (and who do not have SLE). Treatment with rest and low-dose aspirin and heparin (an injected blood-thinning agent) may help.

Thyroid disease

Thyroid disease is not common in pregnant women as in most cases both an underactive or overactive thyroid gland interferes with menstruation, making conception unlikely.

Around 0.5 per cent of pregnant women are hyperthyroid (overactive thyroid). They tend to produce low-birth-weight babies who are born prematurely.

Hypothyroidism (underactive thyroid) is even rarer during pregnancy. It often causes early miscarriage as the developing foetus relies on its mother's thyroid activity until its own thyroid gland develops.

Women with controlled thyroid problems (i.e. on regular medication) are no more likely to have a miscarriage than euthyroid (normal thyroid) women.

Epilepsy

Most women who suffer from epilepsy are more prone to seizures during pregnancy than at any other time. This is because of the hormonal and metabolic changes that occur during pregnancy – and because medication is often modified before pregnancy. Folate supplements also interfere with some anti-epileptic drugs, increasing the risk of a fit (see pages 78 and 169).

Unfortunately, a prolonged *grand mal* fit can result in a miscarriage by interfering with the foetal supply of oxygenated blood.

Epileptic women on medication can be reassured that they have a better than 90 per cent chance of producing a normal child. Preconceptual care is important, however, especially with regard to your nutrient intake. Specialist advice is essential to help you balance your folate and anti-epileptic drug dosage.

Maternal disease associated with pregnancy itself

Excessive morning sickness (hyperemesis gravidarum) during the first three months of pregnancy can cause dehydration and severe electrolyte disturbances. The acid balance of the body becomes abnormal and poisons known as ketones build up in the blood. These result from the body burning fat for energy in the absence of any dietary carbohydrate.

For all the above reasons, excessive morning sickness is potentially harmful to the foetus and in extreme cases may lead to miscarriage. If vomiting is excessive, always seek medical attention. Admission to hospital for drip-feeding and rehydration is sometimes necessary.

Women who develop gestational diabetes, high blood pressure and pre-eclampsia during pregnancy are more likely to suffer late miscarriage or pre-term delivery. Unfortunately, these problems cannot be predicted accurately in advance, hence the need for regular antenatal screening in all pregnant women. If you have had problems in a previous pregnancy, pre-conceptual care and regular monitoring are essential for any future pregnancies.

Urinary tract infections are relatively common in pregnancy. High levels of progesterone hormone relax the smooth muscle walls of the uro-genital tract, allowing easier access for pathogens (organisms causing disease), and also dampen the natural immunological response to infection.

If you experience any urinary symptoms during pregnancy (burning or stinging on passing water, frequency of running to the toilet, low back ache, blood in the urine) seek medical advance sooner rather than later. Untreated urinary tract infections can lead to abdominal pain and threatened miscarriage. Chronic (long-term) low-grade infection can lead to nutrient deficiencies, especially of vitamin B complex. For this reason, it is worth having a sample of urine checked for infection during your pre-conceptual care programme.

Maternal anatomical abnormalities

Anatomical abnormalities of the female genital tract – e.g. a split (septate) uterus with two cavities, a double uterus, an incompetent cervix – can all result in miscarriage. They are relatively uncommon, with an incidence of around 1 in 700 women. Anatomical abnormalities are usually not picked up until investigations are performed for recurrent miscarriage.

An incompetent cervix is essentially too weak to hold the womb closed after the third month of pregnancy. This is easily overcome by inserting a strong stitch around the cervix to hold it closed artificially. This stitch must be removed at around 37 weeks' gestation, or earlier if labour is premature.

Immunological incompatibility between the foetus and the mother

It is now thought that miscarriage is often caused by an immunological incompatibility between the mother and her baby.

The foetus contains cells with genetic markers derived from its father. In effect, the foetus is acting like a transplant of foreign tissue (see page 246).

In any circumstance apart from pregnancy these foreign markers would trigger a violent immunological reaction similar to that seen when transplanted organs are rejected. In some cases of recurrent miscarriage, this may be what is happening.

In exciting new research, trials are taking place to desensitise women to their husbands' antigens. White blood cells are extracted from the father and injected into the mother and this has already proved successful.

Drugs

All drugs, including alcohol, those bought over the counter, those prescribed by doctors and illicit, recreational drugs, are best avoided during the pre-conceptual care period and throughout pregnancy.

Many drugs are linked with early miscarriage or foetal abnormality. Only essential prescribed drugs should be continued and then only after informing the prescribing doctor that you are intending to try for a pregnancy (see page 168).

Recurrent miscarriage

In 95 per cent of cases, spontaneous miscarriage is caused by a non-recurring factor and the prognosis is excellent for carrying a future pregnancy to term. Recurrent, or habitual, miscarriage is diagnosed when three consecutive pregnancies end in spontaneous abortion. The incidence is low, with a risk of 0.4 per cent.

Women suffering from recurrent miscarriage should always be investigated. The cause may not be found, but can include many of the conditions discussed above, e.g. nutrient deficiencies, toxins, foetal structural or genetic abnormalities, maternal uterine or cervical abnormalities, maternal systemic illnesses and immuno-logical incompatibilities.

New research may lead to the diagnosis of previously unrecognised conditions such as high LH levels or anti-phospholipid antibodies (see pages 261 and 262).

In up to 5 per cent of couples, recurrent miscarriage is caused by an abnormal chromosome pattern in one parent. The parent appears well but the abnormality renders them essentially subfertile.

Genetic analysis and counselling is therefore an important part of the investigative process when recurrent miscarriage occurs (see page 180).

What to do if you have previously suffered a miscarriage

Women who have suffered one or two miscarriages are advised to follow a pre-conceptual care programme with their partner which ensures an adequate nutritional intake. The woman should rest and not try for another pregnancy until at least three or four months have elapsed.

In some women, hair analysis to detect mineral deficiencies or toxic compounds has proved useful to correct imbalances. This is advocated by the pre-conceptual care charity Foresight, whose address is given on page 272.

Foresight also offers tests to look for allergies which may be linked to recurrent miscarriage. Foresight say that of the women they have counselled and advised on pre-conceptual care, only one in 31 goes on to miscarry, compared with a national average of one in 2.7 women. This is an order of magnitude difference which would seem to prove their success.

Unfortunately, new research suggests that recurrent pregnancy loss may increase the risk of the next child born having a birth defect. The risk of a serious birth defect was found to increase from under 3 per cent in infants whose mother had no prior pregnancy loss to just over 4 per cent in infants whose mother had had three or more previous miscarriages.

This finding is not unexpected, given that recurrent miscarriage may be caused by genetic abnormalities or by nutrient deficiencies such as folate or vitamin B12.

All women with pre-existing medical conditions should certainly consult a specialist for advice during their pre-conceptual care programme.

Pre-conceptual testing for risk of miscarriage

A British team are developing a system of tests which will show whether hostile substances in maternal blood (e.g. antibodies, pollutants, pesticides, drugs, etc.) are likely to increase the risk of miscarriage *before* conception has occurred.

By incubating a piece of non-human embryonic tissue in the presence of the future mother's serum (blood minus the blood cells), they can predict which women are capable of supporting pregnancy.

Results so far are hopeful in that they give the expected result when tested on groups with known chances of fertility:

- Serum from women taking chemotherapy could not support normal development of embryonic tissue.
- Serum from women who had previously had a child with a neural tube defect could not support embryonic development in 60 per cent of cases.
- In women who had previously had one miscarriage, the serum from 30 per cent could not support embryonic development.

All the above results are as expected. The researchers now hope to perfect the test to identify women in whom a problem exists. The limitation of the test is that it cannot predict the 30 per cent of potential miscarriers in whom anatomical or one-off genetic abnormalities will cause problems during future pregnancy.

The future

It may not seem like it, but having a miscarriage does offer some hope. By proving that conception is possible, a miscarriage is one step further on than the misery felt by couples who suffer infertility and for whom conception seems an unobtainable goal.

In most cases, a woman who has suffered two consecutive miscarriages still has a 70 per cent chance of a future pregnancy continuing to the successful delivery of a child. Even women who have suffered six or more miscarriages still have a 50 per cent chance of a future successful pregnancy, unless a specific, recurring abnormality is diagnosed.

By following a pre-conceptual care programme, the message is very much one of hope.

Appendix

Table of simple advice for both partners

Start at least three months before trying to conceive – and preferably six.

- Decide on a method of contraception.
- Eat organic whole foods where possible.
- Avoid tinned foods, processed foods and excess salt.
- Eliminate all dietary additives.
- Wash all vegetables, fruit and salad stuff thoroughly.
- Eat five portions of fruit or veg per day.
- Eat 30 g nuts, seeds or pulses per day.
- Reduce fat intake to below 30 per cent of energy intake.
- Reduce saturated fat intake to less than 10 per cent of total calories.
- Eat at least 50 per cent of your energy as complex carbohydrate (wholewheat pasta, potatoes, wholemeal bread, brown rice, etc.).
- Obtain 25 g to 30 g of fibre per day.
- Cut down on red meat.
- Eat more fish, especially fresh oily fish at least twice a week.
- Eat fresh foods, organically grown where possible, rather than tinned, pre-packed or processed foods.
- Reduce intake of salt and refined sugar.
- Garlic, yoghurt, bananas and pectin-containing fruits help to

reduce absorption of dietary toxins.
- Both partners should stop smoking. Smokers are only half as fertile as non-smokers.
- Cut out alcohol – 40 per cent of infertility is linked to moderate alcohol intake.
- Decrease your consumption of caffeine ideally to no more than three cups of tea and coffee per day.
- Take appropriate multi-nutrient supplements according to your dietary intake.
- Lose any excess weight.
- Improve your general fitness through exercise.
- Learn to beat stress with relaxation techniques and try therapies such as aromatherapy, homeopathy, acupuncture.
- Avoid using aluminium kitchenware and foil.
- Eliminate all non-essential drugs.
- Consider either:
  - having your water supply analysed for toxic metals
  - using a water filter, or
  - using bottled mineral water.
- Avoid heavy traffic and inhaling exhaust fumes.

Additional pre-conceptual care advice for women

- Take supplements of folate and vitamin B12.
- Consider taking multi-vitamin and mineral supplements depending on your dietary intake.
- Ensure an adequate intake of antioxidant vitamins and minerals – especially vitamin C, E, betacarotene, zinc, selenium, chromium and manganese.
- Avoid listeria-risk foods.
- Avoid raw eggs and products.
- Take anti-toxoplasmosis precautions.
- Consider hair mineral analysis.
- Only have white dental fillings fitted.

Additional pre-conceptual advice for men

Start at least 100 days before trying to conceive.

- Wear loose cotton boxer shorts.
- Consider daily cold water douching of the testicles.
- Avoid hot baths.
- Consider taking supplements of vitamins C, E, betacarotene and the mineral zinc.

Useful addresses

UK

Please send a stamped, self-addressed envelope if writing to any organisation for information leaflets.

Foresight
28 The Paddock
Godalming
Surrey GU7 1XD
Tel: 01483 427839
www.foresight-preconception.org.uk
Advice on pre-conceptual care, recurrent miscarriage, infertility. Private general health checks. Dietary advice. Leaflets, books.

Maternity Alliance
Third Floor West
Northburgh Street
London EC1V 0AY
Tel: 020 7490 7639
www.maternityalliance.org.uk
Information on pre-conceptual care, maternity rights and benefits. Leaflets.

Well woman and gynaecology clinics
Marie Stopes
153–157 Cleveland Street
London W1T 6QW

Tel: 020 7574 7400
www.mariestopes.org.uk

British Pregnancy Advisory Service
Austy Manor
Wootton Wawen
Solihull
West Midlands B95 6BX
Tel: 08457 304030
www.bpas.org
Advice and counselling on termination, female sterilisation and
vasectomy. Leaflets.

Brook (formerly Brook Advisory Centres)
421 Highgate Studios
53–79 Highgate Road
London NW5 1TL
Tel: 020 7284 6040
www.brook.org.uk
Advice and information on contraception. Pregnancy testing and
counselling. Leaflets, booklets.

Family Planning Association (fpa)
2–12 Pentonville Road
London N1 9FP
Tel: 0845 310 1334
www.fpa.org.uk

LIFE
Life House
Newbold Terrace
Leamington Spa
Warwickshire CV32 4EA
Tel: 01926 311667
www.lifeuk.org
A charity offering information and advice on all aspects of
pregnancy, abortion, stillbirth and miscarriage.

Miscarriage Association
Clayton Hospital
Northgate
Wakefield
West Yorkshire WF1 3JS
Tel: 01924 200799
www.miscarriageassociation.org.uk
Support and advice to women and families experiencing
miscarriages. Leaflets, newsletters.

National Childbirth Trust (NCT)
Alexandra House
Oldham Terrace
London W3 6NH
Tel: 0870 444 8707
www.nctpregnancyandbabycare.com
Information, counselling and support during pregnancy,
childbirth and early parenthood. Antenatal classes. Leaflets,
booklets.

WellBeing
27 Sussex Place
Regent's Park
London NW1 4SP
Tel: 020 7772 6400
www.wellbeing.org.uk
Funds medical research for better health of women and babies.
Leaflets and newsletter.

Women's Health
Information Centre
52 Featherstone Street
London EC1Y 8RT
Tel: 0845 125 5254
www.womenshealthlondon.org.uk
See also PID network below.

Diet

Sainsburys/WellBeing Eating for Pregnancy
Helpline: 0114 242 4084

The Vegetarian Society
Parkdale
Dunham Road
Altrincham
Cheshire
WA14 4QG
Tel: 0161 925 2000
www.vegsoc.org

Infections

Congenital CMV Association
69 The Leasowes
Ford
Shrewsbury
Shropshire SY5 9LU
Tel: 01743 850055
Information, advice and support to families with a child affected
by cytomegolovirus. Leaflets, newsletter.

Herpes Viruses Association
39–41 North Road
London N7 9DP
Helpline: 0207 609 9061
www.herpes.org.uk
Information and advice to sufferers (please send an SAE).

National AIDS Helpline
Tel: 0800 567 123
Provides free, confidential information and advice on HIV and
AIDS 24 hours a day, seven days a week.

Pelvic Inflammatory Disease Network
Women's Health
c/o 52 Featherstone Street
London EC1Y 8RT
Tel: 0845 125 5254
www.womenshealthlondon.org.uk
Information about PID. Newsletter, leaflets, meetings.

Toxoplasmosis Trust
c/o Tommys Campaign
1 Kennington Road
London SE1 7RR
Tel: 020 7620 0188
www.tommys.org
Advice and support to sufferers and their families. Advice on
prevention of toxoplasmosis during pregnancy. Leaflets,
newsletter, support network.

Infertility

Child
Charter House
43 St Leonard's Road
Bexhill-on-Sea
East Sussex TN40 1JA
Tel: 01424 732361
www.child.org.uk
Advice and support to those having difficulty conceiving.
Promotes research into infertility.

British Pregnancy Advisory Service
Austy Manor
Wootton Wawen
Solihull, West Midlands B95 6BX
Tel: 08457 304030
www.bpas.org
Donor insemination service. Also advice and medical help for
unwanted pregnancy, emergency contraception and sterilisation.

Miscellaneous

Alcohol Concern
Waterbridge House
32–36 Loman Street
London SE1 0EE
Tel: 020 7928 7377
www.alcoholconcern.org.uk
Help and advice for those worried about their drinking. Leaflets,
counselling.

Association for Spina Bifida and Hydrocephalus
ASBAH House
42 Park Road
Peterborough PE1 2UQ
Tel: 01733 555988
www.asbah.org
Advice, support and welfare services to help new parents with an
affected child. Leaflets, booklets, newsletter.

Cleft Lip and Palate Association (CLAPA)
235–237 Finchley Road
London NW3 6LS
Tel: 020 7431 0033
www.clapa.com

Cystic Fibrosis Trust
11 London Road
Bromley
Kent BR1 1BY
Tel: 020 8464 7211
www.cftrust.org.uk

Down's Syndrome Association
155 Mitcham Road
London SW17 9PG
Tel: 020 8682 4001

www.downs-syndrome.org.uk
Information, advice and support for families with a member
affected by Down's syndrome. Leaflets, booklets, newsletter.

Eating Disorders Association
First Floor
Wensum House
103 Prince of Wales Road
Norwich NR1 1DW
www.edauk.com
Tel: 01603 664 915

Genetic Interest Group
Unit 4D, Leroy House
436 Essex Road
London N1 3QP
Tel: 020 7704 3141
www.gig.org.uk
Information about genetic disorders. Factsheet, newsletter.

QUIT
Ground Floor
211 Old Street
London EC1V 9NR
Smokers' Quitline: 0800 002200
www.quit.org.uk
Advice and counselling on giving up smoking.

Scope
Cerebral Palsy Helpline
PO Box 833
Milton Keynes MK12 5NY
Tel: 0808 800 3333
www.scope.org.uk

Support after Termination of Pregnancy for Abnormality
now ARC (Antenatal Results and Choices)
73 Charlotte Street
London W1T 4PN
Tel: 020 7631 0285
www.arc-uk.org
Support to parents when an abnormality is detected during
pregnancy.

Australia – ACT

Pregnancy and contraception
The Australian Council of Natural Family Planning Inc.
36 Fergusson Street
PO Box 529
Forestville
NSW 2087
Tel: 09 452 5244

Family Planning Association ACT
Suite 4
Level 1
Construction House
Northbourne Avenue
Turner
ACT 2602
Tel: 06 230 5255

Family Planning Australia
PO Box 256
Lyneham
ACT 2602

Pregnancy Advisory Service
Childers Street
Canberra City
ACT 2601
Tel: 06 248 6222

Pregnancy Support Service ACT Inc
PO Box 476
Civic Square
ACT 2608
Tel: 06 249 1779

SANDS (Stillbirth And Neonatal Death Support)
Suite 208
901 White Horse Road
Boxhill
VICTORIA 3128
Tel: 03 9899 0217

Diet

Local Community Health Centres
Listed under 'Health' in the *White Pages*.

Public Hospital Nutrition Departments
Woden Valley Hospital: 06 244 2222
Calvary Hospital: 06 201 6111

Infections

AIDS Action Council
Tel: 06 257 2855

AIDS Reference Centre
Tel: 06 244 2184

Miscellaneous

Alcohol and Drug Information Service
Tel: 06 205 4545

Calvary Hospital
Antenatal classes: 06 201 6030

Canberra Women's Health Centre
Tel: 06 286 2043

Childbirth Education Association
Tel: 08 539 7188

Drug Referral Information Centre
Tel: 06 248 7677

Family Care Centre
Tel: 06 205 1630

Homebirth Canberra Inc
Tel: 06 287 2330

QUITS
Tel: 06 282 3452
(Stop smoking programme.)

Woden Valley Hospital
Birth Centre: 06 244 3145
Parent Education Unit: 06 244 3136
Pre-Admission Antenatal Clinic: 06 244 3466

Australian states

New South Wales
Leichhardt Women's Health Centre
Tel: 09 560 3011

Northern Territory
Darwin Women's Information Centre
Tel: 08 951 5880

Queensland
Brisbane Women's Health Centre
Tel: 07 839 9988

South Australia
Adelaide Women's Health Centre
Tel: 08 267 5366

Tasmania
Hobart Women's Health Centre
Tel: 02 313 212

Victoria
Healthsharing Women
Tel: 03 9760 0669

Western Australia
Women's Health Care House
Tel: 09 227 8122

Canada

Planned Parenthood Federation Canada
1 Nicholas Street
Suite 430
Ottowa
Ontario K1N 7B7
Tel: 0101 613 241 4474

New Zealand

New Zealand Family Planning Association
Level 6
Southmark House
203–209 Willis Street
PO Box 11 515
Wellington
Tel: (04) 384 4349
Fax: (04) 382 8356

South Africa

Association for Dietetics
PO Box 4309
Randburg 2125

Index

ALSO AVAILABLE
FROM VERMILION

☐ Alternative Infertility Treatments	0091815428	£8.99
☐ Birth and Beyond	0091856949	£17.99
☐ From Conception to Birth	0091887682	£25.00
☐ Taking Charge of Your Fertility	0091887585	£14.99
☐ The New Contented Little Baby Book	0091882338	£9.99
☐ The Pilates Pregnancy	0091882893	£10.99

FREE POST AND PACKING
Overseas customers allow £2.00 per paperback

BY PHONE: 01624 677237

BY POST: Random House Books
c/o Bookpost
PO Box 29
Douglas
Isle of Man, IM99 1BQ

BY FAX: 01624 670923

BY EMAIL: bookshop@enterprise.net

Cheques (payable to Bookpost) and
credit cards accepted

Prices and availability subject to change without notice.
Allow 28 days for delivery.
When placing your order, please mention if you do not wish
to receive any additional information.

www.randomhouse.co.uk